the

2

day diet

Diet two days a week.

Eat the Mediterranean way for five.

Dr. Michelle Harvie and Professor Tony Howell

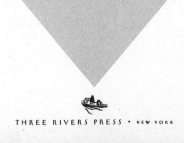

THREE RIVERS PRESS • NEW YORK

*This book is dedicated to four special
people who constantly inspire and
support me: my parents, Mary
and Terry Harvie; my wonderful
partner, Mark Garrod; and my
colleague and friend, Tony Howell.*
– Dr. Michelle Harvie

*This book is dedicated
to my wife, Shelagh, for
her patience and support.*
– Prof. Tony Howell

contents

Originally published in paperback in Great Britain by Vermilion, an imprint of Ebury Publishing, a Random House Group Company, London.

All recipes by Kate Santon with the exception of the recipes on pages 183, 184, 186–187, 192–193, 198, 200–201, 209–211, 215–216, 221–224, 226–228, 300 by Emily Jonzen

Library of Congress Cataloging-in-Publication Data
Harvie, Michelle.
    The 2-day diet : diet two days a week, eat the Mediterranean way for five / Dr. Michelle Harvie and Prof. Tony Howell.
        pages cm
    1. Reducing diets—Recipes.   2. Weight loss.   3. Diet—Mediterranean Region.
4. Diet therapy—Mediterranean Region.   I. Howell, Tony (Professor)   II. Title.
III. Title: Two day diet.
    RM222.2.H317 2013
    613.2'5—dc23   2013012516

ISBN 978-0-804-13840-6
eISBN 978-0-804-13841-3

All author proceeds from the sale of this book will go to Genesis Breast Cancer Prevention (Registered charity number 1109839).

Printed in the United States of America

10 9 8 7 6 5 4 3 2 1

First American Edition

introduction

It won't come as a surprise to anyone reading this that we are getting fatter. Rates of obesity have reached epidemic proportions, and worldwide there are now more overweight people than those who are a healthy weight. Despite massive government investment in healthy eating campaigns and any number of different diets promising effective weight loss, the number of us who are overweight just keeps rising.

But let's be clear, losing weight, even avoiding gaining it, is hard work in today's world. We are genetically programmed for an environment where food supplies are scarce and irregular, and we have to expend huge amounts of energy hunting it down—not for a world where food is available 24/7, we drive everywhere, and are constantly tempted by supersized portions. With all this working against us it's hardly surprising that obesity rates keep rising. Losing weight is a struggle for anyone, however determined they are.

Our day-to-day contact with people desperate to lose weight means that we understand just how hard dieting can be and the frustration and heartache that come when you lose weight . . . then pile it back on. We also know how dangerous extra weight can be for your health. Our research is mainly focused on how excess weight increases the risk of cancer, but extra weight also contributes to heart disease, diabetes, and dementia. As scientists with a commitment not just to our patients but also to improving the nation's health, we decided it was time to develop a research-based diet that would offer a different way to lose weight and keep it off.

With so many different diets available, can The 2-Day Diet really make a difference? We believe that it can. The 2-Day Diet is designed to help you make the right choices, lose weight, change your habits, and actively improve your health without leaving you feeling deprived. Our work with serial dieters has shown that this unique approach offers a real alternative for anyone who struggles to stick to a conventional diet. We were so impressed by the positive results of The 2-Day Diet that we wanted to make it available to everyone who is struggling—or who has struggled—to lose weight. The 2-Day Diet has paved the way to a slimmer, healthier future for many of our dieters. We hope it will do the same for you.

1

why The 2-Day Diet works

If you are someone who has tried, and failed, to lose weight, or you've shed the extra pounds only to pile them back on again—this is the book for you. The 2-Day Diet is a brand new, research-based approach to weight loss that can work for you whether you've been struggling with your weight for years or have only just made the decision to lose weight. The 2-Day Diet is simple: you diet for just two consecutive days a week and eat normally for the other five days.

I have never dieted and successfully kept the weight off —before I tried The 2-Day Diet. In fact, I have always regained the weight and then usually extra, too. The 2-Day Diet is different—it's a lifestyle change that I can actually live with. —Marie, 33

We have become used to diet experts telling us that if we want to lose weight, there are strict rules that we must follow every day. The 2-Day Diet approach turns all of that theory on its head. It's flexible, it's easy to follow, and it will make you rethink your approach to dieting and find a different way to lose your unwanted pounds.

The idea of escaping the day-in, day-out restriction of a seven-day diet regime—dieting for just two days a week and eating normally for the other five days and still losing weight—probably sounds too good to be true. But it's not: our weight-loss research over the last 17 years with dieters, many of them serial dieters, shows that this new approach really can work, even when everything else has failed. The 2-Day Diet has been designed by research dietitian Dr. Michelle Harvie, and, as well as delivering healthy, sustainable weight loss, The 2-Day Diet is nutritionally balanced to meet all your body's needs.

Dieting on the two days was much easier than I had expected. I also found that I was much more mindful of my eating over the five normal eating days—I didn't want to undo all that good work! —Lizzie, 24

Warning

You should not attempt The 2-Day Diet if you are a child, a teenager, pregnant, breast-feeding, suffering from depression, or have an eating disorder. The moderately high levels of protein in this diet may pose problems for anyone with kidney disease or anyone at risk of kidney disease. If you have diabetes or any other medical condition, or if you are taking medication, seek advice from your doctor before embarking on any diet and exercise program.

If you are overweight, your main motivation for dieting may be to improve your self-esteem by regaining your true figure. You will lose weight on The 2-Day Diet, but you will also improve your health, protect yourself against disease, and boost your energy levels. Research shows that losing even a small amount of excess weight (5 to 10 percent of your body weight) can help reduce your risk of diseases such as type 2 diabetes, heart disease, and some cancers. What's more, there's evidence to show that losing weight with The 2-Day Diet has the potential to have even greater health benefits than those gained by using a daily dieting weight-loss plan, as we will explain later.

The diet trap

In theory, losing weight should be easy. Eat less, move around more, and the pounds should simply melt away. In practice, losing weight can be anything but easy. You might be able to lose a few pounds in the short term, but they soon creep back on again. Despite major public health campaigns and millions of dollars spent each year on diet products, the number of people who are overweight keeps on rising in almost all parts of the world, but particularly in the USA and UK. In 2010, 64 percent of American women and 74 percent of men were overweight. These figures occur alongside reports estimating that 108 million people in the USA follow weight-loss diets each year, spending $20 billion per annum on diet books, diet drugs and weight-loss surgery. A 2007 MORI survey found that the average UK woman spends 31 years of her life on a diet, yet British women are now the heaviest in Europe. British men don't fare much better—66 percent are now overweight, positioning them as the second-heaviest in Europe. It's clearly time for a new approach.

I can see and feel the weight loss, so I feel better
about myself. I don't feel so tired—I have so much
more energy in the evenings. —Jane, 32

The story behind The 2-Day Diet

Our search for a different way to lose weight was driven by our work over nearly two decades with women diagnosed with, or at high risk from, breast cancer. We knew from our research and work done elsewhere that while being overweight significantly increases women's risk of developing breast cancer, losing weight—even as little as 10 lb (4.5 kg)—can cut that risk by between 25 and 40 percent, compared with women who continue to gain weight, which is the norm.[1] The problem is that losing weight—and keeping it off—is extraordinarily difficult. Typically the dieters we worked with had already made between three and five serious attempts to lose weight. However motivated they were and however hard they tried, less than half of them managed to shed the weight needed to reduce their risk. Many enjoyed amazing short-term success and displayed extraordinary willpower and determination, but, sadly, for most, the weight loss didn't last.

CASE STUDY: Anne

Anne's story is typical. Anne was desperate to lose weight, knowing that it was increasing her risk of developing the breast cancer that had already affected her mother, aunt, and cousin, and her chance of developing type 2 diabetes, which had affected her father's side of the family. She had previously managed to lose 42 lbs (19 kg) at a weight-loss group over a period of five months. This must have involved her eating 900 calories less than she normally ate each day for five months—133,000 fewer calories in all! However, unfortunately, after all this effort, she regained most of the weight within four months.

Typically people stick with a diet for three to six months and lose around 14 lbs (6.4 kg) in weight. The majority of people—80 percent—then put most of the weight back on again, while the remaining 20 percent regain some weight but remain 8–12 lbs (3.6–5.4 kg) lighter than their pre-diet weight.[2]

So dieting isn't entirely in vain, since it can prevent you from gaining even more weight in the longer term. However, the process of constantly losing and regaining weight is demoralizing, can lower your self-esteem, and can undermine subsequent attempts to lose weight. As many dieters are only too aware, dieting is a constant drudge.

Thanks to The 2-Day Diet I feel less sluggish, less bloated, less tired after exercise, much healthier, and my clothes now fit more comfortably. —Honor, 45

The size of the problem

- From 1950–1960 33 percent of adults in the US were overweight (defined as a BMI of 25 or higher) and 9.7 percent were classified as obese (with a BMI of 30 or higher). The latest figures show that 6 percent of women are overweight and 36 percent obese, while 74 percent of men are overweight with 36 percent obese.[3] Very roughly you can think of it this way: one-third of us are a healthy weight, one-third are overweight, and one-third obese.

- The US government currently spends as much as $147 million each year on weight-related problems, which could rise to $334 billion a year by 2018.
- A recent study by Duke University Medical Center reported that overweight workers miss 12 times more work days than non-obese workers.[4]
- In 2006, the United Nations announced that for the first time, the number of overweight people in the world exceeded those who were undernourished, with more than 1.3 billion people overweight and 800 million underweight.

Why diet for just two days a week?

Our initial studies between 1995 and 2005 used the conventional dieting approach and asked our Dieters to cut down calories on all seven days of the week. It became clear that many struggled with this standard approach, as they found themselves constantly having to think about their diet and what they were eating. By 2005, intriguing evidence of "intermittent dieting," where calories are restricted for some days of the week, with a normal dietary intake for the other days, had started to emerge from scientists working in the fields of cancer and dementia. Papers published in 2002 and 2003 described how animals in the laboratory that were placed on intermittent diets developed significantly fewer cancers and less dementia than their counterparts that were following standard daily restricted diets.[5,6] Although these original studies involved animals rather than people, the findings got us thinking. Most diets expect people to cut calories every day of the week, typically eating 25 percent fewer calories each day and sticking to that regime. But what would happen if you did most of your dieting during two strictly observed days each week when you had around 70 percent fewer calories on these two days rather than trying to cut down by the usual 25 percent every day? Dieting for just two days each week could be a relief from the chore of having to diet every single day, which so many people struggle with. At the same time, two days is long enough to reduce your overall weekly calories, retrain your eating habits, and, crucially, it seemed to have the potential to be more achievable. Would this approach be easier to follow than a daily diet? Could it be a better and more effective way to lose weight?

So back in 2006 we started researching two-day diets with funding from Genesis Breast Cancer Prevention and two other cancer charities (Breast Cancer Campaign and the World Cancer Research Fund), all of whom wanted to find more effective weight-loss approaches to help reduce cancer risk.

The 2-Day Diet is a much more straightforward diet than any other I've been on. The two days "on" are easy to deal with if you put in a tiny amount of planning, and doing it two days a week really makes you respect food on the days you aren't doing it. I lost 5 lb (2 kg) in the first 10 days and I don't have that "I'm on a diet" feeling.
—Matt, 41

Our first 2-Day Diet
The first 2-Day Diet we devised included two days of 650-calorie intake that only permitted milk, yogurt, fruit, vegetables, and unlimited low-calorie drinks such as water, tea, coffee, and diet drinks. The 650-calorie days were care-

fully designed to ensure that the Dieters met their nutritional requirements. Our 2-Day Dieters followed this diet for two consecutive days each week, eating a healthy Mediterranean diet (see page 70) for the other five days. They were then compared with a group of dieters who were asked to reduce their overall calorie intake by the same amount as the 2-Day Dieters, but by eating a standard, reduced-food intake every day of the week. A total of 107 women took part.

What we learned

We were encouraged by the results from this study. There was some evidence that, although the results were not substantially different from standard daily dieting, a two-day approach might be easier for some people to follow and have the potential for weight loss.

After six months, 54 percent of the 2-Day Dieters and 51 percent of the daily dieters were successful and had lost at least 5 percent of their weight. The 2-Day Dieters who stuck with the Diet for six months lost, on average, 17 lb (7.7 kg) of weight, of which 13¼ lb (6 kg) was fat, as well as 3 in (7.6 cm) from their waists, and 2⅓ in (6 cm) from their hips and bust. Some lost far more, with weight losses of 46 lb (21 kg) and dropping at least three clothes sizes. For daily dieters, on average there was a 13 lb 9 oz (6.3 kg) weight loss, a 10 lb 8 oz (4.9 kg) loss of fat, and a loss of 2 in (5 cm) from the waist and bust.

Moreover, two-day dieting appeared to deliver greater health benefits than the daily diet. Both approaches were beneficial, but our 2-Day Dieters had a 25 percent greater improvement in their insulin function than the daily dieters when we measured this five days after their restriction. They had a further 25 percent reduction during and on the morning immediately after their two restricted days.[7] Insulin plays a vital role in regulating sugar levels in the body. Poor insulin function is a serious problem in modern life and is at the root of many weight-related diseases, such as type 2 diabetes, heart disease, some cancers, and possibly dementia. A large waist measurement is also associated with a greater risk of many of these diseases, and our 2-Day Dieters also lost proportionately more weight from the waist than the seven-day dieters.

The intermittent diet approach could even be used for weight maintenance. Our 2-Day Dieters who lost weight switched to just one restricted day a week, kept the weight off, and maintained the health benefits for the 15 months of the study—importantly, they maintained the reductions in insulin and cholesterol they had achieved with the diet.

Our new, improved 2-Day Diet

Using the lessons we had learned throughout our original diet research, we developed The 2-Day Diet, which forms the focus of this book.

Predictably the main downside of our original 2-Day Diet was that the food choices were so limited. Many of the Dieters on the trial found that only being able to have milk, yogurt, fruit, and vegetables was hard to stick to, and only one-third of them were still following the diet by the end of a year. But we were so encouraged by the findings from our early research that we improved the Diet to include a greater variety of foods and included more protein foods to make the Diet more satisfying, filling, and easier to maintain long-term. Once again we tested The 2-Day Diet with two groups of women: one group doing the new, improved 2-Day Diet, the other a standard daily diet.

The feedback on the new, improved 2-Day Diet was even more impressive. Our most recent study, which followed

women over three months' dieting and a month's maintenance found that six out of 10 women who set out to follow the
Diet were successful, losing at least 10 lb (4.5 kg), compared
with only four out of 10 following a standard daily diet.[8]
Weight loss in this three-month study was slightly lower than
our previous six-month dieters as this was a shorter spell of
dieting. However, the weight loss we achieved was particularly
encouraging as these Dieters were older, heavier, and many had
long-term weight and health problems.

The Dieters who managed to do at least 85 percent of their
two restricted days during the study (i.e., 20 out of their 24
days over three months) had the greatest rewards. On average they lost almost 14 lb (6.4 kg), over 10 lb (4.5 kg) of it
fat, lost 2 in (5 cm) from the waist and hips, and dropped a
clothes size. Again, some lost far more weight—they dropped
two clothes sizes in three months, losing as much as 32 lb
(14.5 kg), 24 lb (10.8 kg) of it fat, just over 4⅓ in (10.9
cm) from the waist and hips, and 3½ in (8.9 cm) from the
bust. As before, our 2-Day Dieters had much greater reductions
in insulin than seven-day dieters five days after their restricted
days, and again they had the bonus of a further reduction of
insulin during the two days when the calorie and carbohydrate
intakes were actually reduced.

How The 2-Day Diet works

The 2-Day Diet provides clear guidelines about what you can
eat on your two restricted "diet" days. You eat foods that are
high in protein, healthy monounsaturated fats (such as nuts),
and fruit and vegetables, which are satisfying and reduce the
feelings of hunger. Feeling fuller obviously makes you less
likely to overeat. The 2-Day Diet is deliberately low in carbohydrates, which appear to make people feel hungrier.[9] On the

other five, unrestricted, days you eat a normal, healthy, Mediterranean-style diet (see page 70).

The 2-Day Diet is designed to be:

▶ Low enough in calories to enable you to lose weight, but without leaving you feeling hungry.

▶ Nutritionally balanced so that all your vitamin, mineral, and protein requirements are met.

▶ Easy to fit into a normal, busy lifestyle.

How is The 2-Day Diet different from other diets?
Cutting down for just two days is easier than cutting down every day.

Overall people found it easier to stick to two strict days than cutting calories every day. Although our seven-day and 2-Day Dieters both started well, with eight in 10 of them sticking to the diets during the first month, the seven-day diet became more of a struggle. After three months, 70 percent of 2-Day Dieters were still following their diet, compared with only 40 percent of the seven-day group.

So why is a stricter regime easier to follow than a less-restricted diet? The answer seems to be precisely because it *is* strict. The 2-Day Diet has clear rules. From discussions with our 2-Day Dieters and previous research we know that as long as the diet is achievable, diets with restricted rules and limited choice can be easier to stick to than healthy-eating, low-calorie diets that have very flexible rules.[10]

In fact, our bodies may even be biologically programmed for this intermittent pattern of eating. The idea of having spells of normal intake and spells of restriction isn't new, and some argue that it mimics the periods of food abundance and scarcity experienced by our hunter-gatherer Paleolithic ancestors, who frequently went for long periods with very little food, interspersed with spells of eating more when food was available and abundant. This is a far cry from today's 24/7 food availability (and the fact that we don't have to hunt for it). Most people in the developed world have unlimited access to as much food as they want around the clock. In fact, many people don't even experience a real overnight fast because they indulge in very late-night eating in front of the TV—perhaps a late snack at 2 a.m., with breakfast only five hours later at 7 a.m.

The 2-Day Diet retrains your eating habits
One reason why dieting is so hard is that it means breaking ingrained eating habits—habits such as regularly consuming more food than we need, eating overly large servings, having too many fatty or sugary foods, or habitual snacking (and often all of these). The 2-Day Diet helps you to change the way you eat. Losing weight is really very simple: it means cutting your overall calories by at least one-quarter and reducing your intake of high-sugar foods and saturated fat. For many people, this is easier said than done. The 2-Day Diet gives you a much-needed break from your normal eating habits each week and helps you to develop vigilance and awareness of what you eat. These are vital skills, which put you on the road to being in control of what you eat and, therefore, your weight.

The 2-Day Diet develops your appreciation of food
Dramatically cutting calories for two days a week helps you to relearn how hunger feels and what a "normal" serving looks like. You will learn to eat more slowly, appreciate smaller amounts, and really enjoy your food on both your two restricted

days and on the five unrestricted days. This will help you to rediscover how much food you really need, rather than the amount you have become used to eating. Our Dieters found that contrasting the two restricted days to their normal intake helped them identify what triggered them to eat—and to over-eat. If you're a serial dieter, you may have become stuck in the low-fat, low-protein, high-carbohydrate pattern of eating, a combination promoted by many mainstream diets. While this approach may work for some, others find it difficult to main-tain a daily low-calorie intake with these regimes, so they often find themselves overeating. The 2-Day Diet will help wean you away from these unhelpful patterns of eating.

The 2-Day Diet boosts your dieting confidence

For two days every week you have the opportunity to learn to resist temptation. This is a key dieting skill that you will need to practice until it becomes a habit. Being restrained on the two restricted days will give you the confidence to master your diet and food cravings and reinforce your desire to be in control of your diet on the other days of the week.

The success of The 2-Day Diet

The 2-Day Diet helps you lose fat rather than muscle

The best diets target fat and preserve muscle. Muscle doesn't just make you look and feel more toned, it's also the key to calorie burning. Even when your muscles are resting, they burn up to seven times as many calories as fat (see below). Dieters who followed the improved 2-Day Diet found that they lost proportionally more fat than the seven-day dieters, with 80 percent of their weight lost as fat compared with 70 percent for the daily diet group. If you follow what is called a "very low calorie diet" (VLCD—around 500–600 cal per day) you can lose only around 60 percent of your weight as fat and 40 percent as muscle. On The 2-Day Diet, for every 14 lb (6.4 kg) you lose, you can expect to lose 11 lb (5 kg) of fat and only 3 lb (1.4 kg) of muscle, compared with 8 lb (3.6 kg) of fat and 6 lb (2.7 kg) of muscle on some VLCDs. Another important point is that staying active while you're on The 2-Day Diet will help maximize your fat loss and limit your muscle loss even further (see page 118).

The 2-Day Diet may help to maintain your metabolic rate

Your metabolic rate, the rate at which your body burns calories, is affected by three things: your weight (the heavier you are, the higher your metabolic rate because your body needs more calories to function); how active you are (active people burn more calories—see Appendix F, page 337); and the amount of muscle you have (the more muscle you have, the higher your metabolic rate because muscle burns seven times more calories than fat). One of the reasons why weight loss slows down when you diet is because your metabolic rate falls, typically by 10 to 15 percent as you lose weight and have less muscle. Because The 2-Day Diet promotes fat loss and minimizes the amount of muscle you lose, it helps to limit the dip in your metabolism. The 2-Day Diet may also help burn a few more calories because of its high protein content—our bodies use 10 times more calories digesting and processing protein than for fat or carbohydrates. Although this doesn't have a major effect—it only burns an extra 65 to 70 calories a day—when you are trying to lose weight, small changes all add up.

You'll see rapid results

Losing weight can be hard work, and dieters need to experience quick rewards so rapid weight loss is key to keeping you on track. There are no quick fixes—fat burning is a complex process, and it's hard to lose more than 4½ lb (2 kg) of fat a week—but you won't need to spend weeks on The 2-Day Diet before you see a difference. The 2-Day Diet performs better than seven-day dieting right from the start and sustains a greater rate of weight loss. Our dieters lost fat about one and a half times as quickly with The 2-Day Diet as with the conventional seven-day diet. After the first month, our 2-Day Dieters lost, on average, 1–3 lb (0.5–1.4 kg) a week, which then slowed slightly. By contrast, the seven-day dieters lost only ½ to 2 lbs (0.3 to 1 kgs) per week.

Our 2-Day Dieters lost more body fat mainly because, overall, they consumed fewer calories; however, they still shed more fat than expected, raising the possibility that they may have experienced a smaller drop in their metabolic rate as their weight decreased than the seven-day dieters—it is an interesting possibility, but one that is as yet unproven.

What happens to your body when you lose weight?

While you are dropping clothes sizes and/or tightening your belt a notch or two and feeling and looking healthier, major changes are taking place in your body. Your blood pressure and levels of harmful blood fats and hormones are all reducing, while favorable ones are increasing. These changes pave the way for a longer, healthier life. Eating too much will cause changes at the most fundamental level inside your body cells, leading to damage that increases your risk of cancer, type 2 diabetes, and even early death. Eating less can halt and even reverse that damage.

How cells work

Your body is made up of millions of cells, and although cells in different areas of your body have different specialist functions—in your brain, heart, and bones, for example—they all work in a similar way. At each cell's heart is a nucleus, the cell's control center, which contains the genes you have inherited (your DNA). Genes are the blueprint for what makes you unique (your hair, eye, and skin color, for example). The activity of the cell is controlled both by the nucleus and by messages sent from within your body, which act on the cell via receptors on its surface. Cells produce their own energy supply and have their own power plants—called mitochondria. Each cell contains around 1,000 of these tiny bean-shaped structures that provide the energy the cell needs to do its essential work. Cells also produce waste products that need to be eliminated, so all cells also have their own waste-disposal units—known as lysosomes—which recycle all the damaged components of the cell.

What happens when you overeat and gain weight?

If you are overfed, then your cells will be too—and overfed cells don't work properly. When you take in more food than you need, levels of the hormones insulin and leptin rise in the body and send a barrage of messages to the cells, telling them to grow and produce lots of new cells. But when cells are putting all their efforts into growth and producing new cells, the lysosomes work less efficiently and the essential maintenance gets neglected, so waste builds up and damage fails to get repaired.

If this happened to your car, it might carry on functioning for a while, but it wouldn't be long before it was off the road. When it happens in your body and you have increasing numbers of poor-quality cells that are not repairing damage and getting rid of waste, it becomes the starting point for many diseases, including cancer.

Overeating is also bad news for your cells' power plants—the mitochondria. They decline in number, become damaged, and stop producing protective antioxidants. Like a worn-out battery, they start to leak harmful "oxidizing" substances, which can damage the cells and surrounding tissues. This damage causes inflammation, which if unchecked can lead to cancer, heart disease, and diabetes.

As well as overfed cells becoming dysfunctional because of the barrage of signals they receive from hormones, overeating actually triggers certain genes in the cell to be switched on and others to be switched off. A recent study found that just five days of feeding healthy young men a high-fat, high-calorie diet caused detrimental changes to their cells by switching on genes associated with inflammation and cancer.[11] By contrast, other studies have shown that eating less and eating the right sort of foods—one example being resveratrol, the protective anti-oxidant found in fruits (especially grapes) and peanuts—can actually reverse these damaging changes and "switch off" the harmful genes.[12]

What is playing out in your cells when you overeat is similar to what happens to your body as you get older—so eating more than your body needs effectively speeds up the clock and ages you prematurely.

Why weight matters

- Being overweight increases the risk of heart disease, stroke, type 2 diabetes, dementia, and more than 12 different cancers, including breast cancer, bowel cancer, and cancers of the esophagus (throat), thyroid gland, kidney, womb, gallbladder, pancreas, malignant melanoma, and cancers of the blood and immune systems, such as leukemia, multiple myeloma, and non-Hodgkins lymphoma.

- People who are overweight are more likely to suffer from arthritis, indigestion, gallstones, stress, anxiety, depression, infertility, and sleep problems.
- Being very overweight (42 lb/19 kg above your healthy weight) is as harmful to health as smoking and can reduce life expectancy by seven years. If you're very overweight and also smoke, it can shorten your life span by 14 years.[13]
- Being overweight limits healthy life expectancy. In the US women live, on average, to the age of 80, but their good health only lasts until age 67, while men live to 75, with good health until the age of 65, often due to weight-related illness.[14]

What happens when you cut your calories?

Restricting your calories and losing weight helps to reverse the cycle of damage described above and gives your cells a spring-cleaning. Levels of insulin and leptin fall quickly (within 24 hours) when we eat less, so their signals that drive the cell to grow reduce, and cells can put more effort into staying in top condition, repairing damage, and removing waste. Damaged old mitochondria are removed and new ones are produced that make more antioxidants, helping to reduce the inflammation in the cells and surrounding tissues. Lowering calorie intake also increases the number of waste-disposal units (lysosomes) and makes them more efficient at waste disposal. These rapid effects within 24 hours of dieting is one of the key reasons The

2-Day Diet has the potential to offer health benefits during the two restricted days each week.

Does this happen with every diet?

If you're overweight, cutting calories and losing weight is likely to produce all the beneficial effects described above. However, The 2-Day Diet, with the two restricted days, in combination with a five-day Mediterranean diet rich in plant chemicals, could be even more beneficial than a regular reduced-calorie diet. The two restricted days help to achieve a 40 percent greater reduction in insulin than a standard calorie-reduced diet. This may be fundamental to the health benefits of The 2-Day Diet, as excess insulin is one of the key drivers for the harmful impact being overweight has on cells and modern chronic diseases. There's also evidence that the lower the intake of calories, the better the waste disposal works, so the low calorie intake on your two restricted days may have extra benefits. Restricting your calories may benefit your brain cells as well as those in the rest of your body. There's evidence from the work of Dr. Mark Mattson, a neuroscientist at the National Institute on Aging in Baltimore, that dramatically reducing your calorie intake for some but not all days of the week could protect against Alzheimer's disease, Parkinson's disease, and other degenerative brain conditions.

Exercise seems to have a similarly beneficial effect on reducing insulin levels, improving waste disposal, and increasing the number of mitochondria. Exercise also has other beneficial effects—when muscles are being used, they produce protective hormones and chemicals. These can help cut your risk of many diseases by improving your body's ability to deal with glucose, reducing inflammation, and lowering levels of growth factors and hormones that are linked with cancer. They can also stimulate cells within the brain for optimal brain health.

What happens to worn-out cells?

Even healthy cells have a limited life and need to be replaced by new cells. This turnover is a natural process, but when your body doesn't work properly because of overeating and inactivity, this gets disrupted so that cells that have completed their useful life persist in the body—these worn-out cells, known as "senescent" cells, are linked to cancer, heart disease, and diabetes. Cutting calories has been shown to reduce the likelihood of these worn-out cells persisting in the body and to ensure that they are eliminated.

CASE STUDY: Gillian

Gillian, 47, started The 2-Day Diet because she knew her weight was creeping up. Although only 14 lb (6.4 kg) overweight, Gillian wanted to get down to a healthy weight and stay there. Gillian wanted a diet that didn't involve special foods or lots of planning, was simple enough to fit into her busy working life, and still meant that she could go out for dinner with friends on the weekend. She did the Diet on her busiest workdays and ate the bulk of her calories in the evening. "Knowing that you're not depriving yourself all week makes this Diet so much easier, and by the time you've finished your two days, you don't feel like eating everything in sight; you just enjoy eating normally. I lost the weight quite easily and kept it off—I often do the Diet for one day a week to keep the weight off."

Your questions answered

Isn't The 2-Day Diet just yo-yo dieting?

Yo-yo dieting and yo-yo weight gain and loss occur when, despite trying to stick to a daily, restricted diet, you end up dipping in and out of it—sometimes dieting and sometimes lapsing.

People often worry that The 2-Day Diet is a type of yo-yo diet, where the Dieter loses weight for two days each week, only to rebound on the days in between. The 2-Day Diet is different, because by carrying out the two-day restriction every week plus maintaining a healthy diet in between, your weight will steadily drop while following the plan.

Why two days?

We wanted to make a departure from the grind of dieting every day. The two days allow long enough to reduce your overall calorie intake and retrain your eating habits, and it may have additional beneficial effects on metabolism and disease risk. It is also achievable.

Do I have to diet for two consecutive days?

We recommend that the two days are done together because many Dieters find the second day as easy, or easier than, the first as they get into the habit of eating less. Doing the two days together also helps to ensure that you actually get around to doing the second day, and it may have additional health benefits because it provides a prolonged period when the body is in a healthier metabolic state (see pages 15–19).

If you struggle to do the two days together each week, two separate days will be fine for weight loss, provided that you actually get around to doing them. In our research, a small number of Dieters—just 5 percent of the total—often did their two days separately, and they still lost weight. You can choose which days of the week work best for you. Many of our Dieters opted for busy working days when they did not have much time to think about missing food, whereas others opted to do them on the weekend when they had more time to be organized. When you do the two days is up to you, but it's probably a good idea to try to keep to the same two days each week to establish a habit that you are more likely to stick to. However, the beauty of just having to diet for two days is that you can swap them, if necessary, to fit into your weekly schedule.

I've heard that just eating once a day can work just as well?

This may be the case if it means that you consume fewer calories overall. However, there are no obvious weight-loss or health benefits from going 24 hours without eating if you eat the same amount of food in one meal as you would have done in a number of meals throughout a day (see page 107).[15]

Don't people just binge on the five unrestricted days?

If you like the idea of dieting for two days but worry about overeating for the rest of the week, you will be pleasantly surprised to hear that our 2-Day Dieters didn't binge on their unrestricted days. In fact, most of them wanted to eat less than they normally did, and this is part of the reason why The 2-Day Diet is successful. A key feature of The 2-Day Diet is that it appears to reset your appetite and retrain your eating behavior for the whole week.

Does it work for everyone?

No diet works for everyone, and this diet is no exception. The success of any diet is mainly due to whether people can follow it and keep it up over time. Our research showed that 60 percent of the Dieters were successful, but 13 percent of those who set out to do The 2-Day Diet had family, work, or other personal issues that prevented them from sticking to it. Thirteen percent of the women who tried it found that they couldn't adhere to it, while a further 14 percent were trying to follow the Diet but had only partial success.

Am I overweight because of my genes?

People often wonder whether their struggle with weight is genetic, and there's been much research over the past five years looking at how one's genetic makeup can affect one's appetite and ability to store fat. However, although there clearly are genetic differences between people (32 weight-related genetic variants have been found so far), these are thought to account for only between 0.5 and 1 percent of the weight variations between different people.[16] So inheriting one of these genes probably means that you are a few pounds heavier than someone who does not. This is a new area of research. In the future we may be able to define the genetic makeup of dieters and identify those who may need extra support with weight loss or a different type of diet, but this is a long way off.

Do my genes make it harder to lose weight?

Although we haven't looked at this in relation to The 2-Day Diet, several recent studies have shown that genes make very little difference in people's ability to lose any weight or the amount they lose. In a recent Spanish study, when dieters followed a 28-week diet and exercise plan, those with a

particular type of gene lost 19 lb (8.6 kg), while those
without the gene lost just 1.5 lb (680 g) more.[17] A recent
Japanese study revealed similar findings. So the take-home
message is that despite having the "weight gene," dieters
were still able to adhere to a diet and exercise regime and to
lose weight.[18]

Do I have to follow The 2-Day Diet—can't I just cut calories for two days?

We don't advise going without food or devising your own two-
day low-calorie diet. The 2-Day Diet has been designed to
keep you feeling as full as possible and to cover your nutritional requirements, with enough protein to limit loss of
muscle mass, which is key to maintaining your metabolic rate
and long-term weight-loss success. If you invent your own
low-calorie diet, you run the risk of its being both difficult to
adhere to and nutritionally incomplete, and it may not have the
beneficial effect on muscle and metabolism.

How will The 2-Day Diet fit in with family life?

It should be easy to fit The 2-Day Diet in with family meals.
On your two restricted days, your family can eat the same as
you, but they can add carbohydrates. For the five unrestricted
days, the healthy Mediterranean-style eating plan (see page 70)
is suitable and beneficial for the health and well-being of the
whole family.

Are there benefits to following The 2-Day Diet if I am already a healthy weight?

The first thing is to check that you really are a healthy weight,
with a healthy level of body fat (see page 30). One in four
people who have a healthy weight on the scales may be

carrying too much fat around their waist. If you have a higher waist measurement than you should (see page 33), you will often also have two or more of the following:

▶ raised level of fat in the blood[a]

▶ raised blood sugar[b]

▶ raised blood pressure[c]

Even if the scales don't say that you're overweight, having weight around your waist puts you at higher risk of heart disease, type 2 diabetes, and possibly certain cancers. If this sounds like you, then losing weight will be beneficial for your health.

If you have a healthy weight and waist measurement, 2-Day Dieting is probably not a good idea, as we don't know the impact of the Diet on individuals who are a healthy weight. However, having one restricted day a week may help you to maintain a healthy weight and to prevent weight gain, especially if you are at a stage of your life when you might be particularly vulnerable to gaining weight (see page 26).

I am a vegetarian—can I still do The 2-Day Diet?

The diet should work just as well for vegetarians as for those who eat meat and fish. The key is to make sure that you include enough protein and don't overload on carbohydrates. There are plenty of filling high-protein vegetarian foods, and you will find plenty of vegetarian recipes for your two restricted days and for the five unrestricted days in chapters 9 and 10.

---

a. Triglycerides: ≥ 150 mg/dl

b. ≥100 mg/dl

c. ≥130/85 mm Hg

Risky times for weight gain

- Recent motherhood, when it is difficult to return to pre-pregnancy weight because of erratic meal patterns and lack of time to exercise. Please note that you should not do The 2-Day Diet if you are breast-feeding. Current guidelines state that once breastfeeding is established, overweight women can cut their calories by 500 cal a day and do 30 minutes of aerobic exercise four days a week to lose around 1 lb (0.5 kg) a week.[19]
- Settling down, cohabiting, and getting married—when women may find themselves eating as much as their partners, despite normally needing far fewer calories.
- Giving up smoking.
- Times of stress and emotional upset.
- Studying or working long hours with many hours sitting at a desk or computer, erratic meal patterns, and often relying on high-calorie snack foods.
- Winter months—when we often crave higher-calorie comfort foods and are less inclined to exercise.
- During the holidays: new research shows that holiday weight gain is about 1 lb (0.5 kg) for the average person, but up to 5 times that for people who are overweight or obese.[20]
- When taking drugs that can cause weight gain, including steroids, oral contraceptives, beta-blockers, and some anti-convulsants and antidepressants.

How much weight will I lose?

The average and maximum weight you can lose in the first three months on The 2-Day Diet is shown below. As you can see, the health benefits occur very rapidly within this first month of dieting.

The drops in cholesterol and blood pressure indicate a reduction in the risk of heart disease of 25–30 percent, and the risk of stroke by 35–40 percent. To maintain these benefits you need to maintain your lower weight and healthy lifestyle behaviors (see chapter 7).

What can be achieved in the first three months of The 2-Day Diet								
	Month 1		Month 2		Month 3		Month 4	
	Average	Max.	Average	Max.	Average	Max.	Average	Max.
Weight	–6 lb (–2.7 kg)	–14½ lb (–6.6 kg)	–4 lb (–1.8 kg)	–12 lb (–5.4 kg)	–3 lb (–1.4 kg)	–8¾ lb (–4.0 kg)	–13 lb (–5.8 kg)	–32 lb (–14.5 kg)
Body fat	–4½ lb (–2 kg)	–11 lb (–5 kg)	–3½ lb (–1.5 kg)	–9½ lb (–4.3 kg)	–1¾ lb (–0.8 kg)	–10 lb (–4.5 kg)	–10 lb (–4.5 kg)	–24 lb (–11 kg)
Waist	–2.6 cm (–1 in)	–6 cm (–2⅓ in)	–2 cm (–¾ in)	–8.5 cm (–3⅓ in)	–1 cm (–⅓ in)	–8 cm (–3 in)	–6 cm (–2⅓ in)	–19 cm (–7½ in)
Insulin change	–10%	–74%	1 to 3 months Average –7% Max. –66%				–12%	–76%
Cholesterol change	–6%	34%	1 to 3 months No change				–6%	–34%
Blood pressure change	–11%	–38%	1 to 3 months No Change				–11%	–40%

Summary

▶ In the USA, 64 percent of American women and 74 percent of men are overweight. The percentage of adults who are overweight in England is one of the highest in Europe and is increasing; 59 percent of women and 66 percent of men are overweight. Despite large amounts of time and money invested in diets, many people struggle to achieve and maintain successful weight loss.

▶ The risk of diseases such as cancer, heart disease, diabetes, and dementia increase with increased weight.

▶ The 2-Day Diet is a new, nutritionally balanced approach to dieting designed to retrain your eating habits, maximize weight loss, and preserve calorie-burning muscle.

▶ The 2-Day Diet involves restricting yourself to eating protein, healthy fats, fruit, and vegetables for two consecutive days each week. For the remaining five unrestricted days, you eat a balanced Mediterranean-style diet.

▶ The 2-Day Diet appears to achieve better and more rapid weight loss, greater health benefits, and, for some Dieters, better long-term success than a standard, every-day restricted-calorie diet.

2

do I need to lose weight?

If your favorite jeans feel a bit too close fitting for comfort or you've found yourself moving up a clothes size or two, the answer to whether you need to lose weight might be obvious. But how can you tell whether your weight gain could actually be harmful to your health? Health problems arise from carrying too much fat—especially if you have fat stored in the wrong places, such as excessive fat in the abdomen or muscles. So just looking in the mirror or standing on the scales may not immediately tell you the answer.

I decided to do the diet because of the way I felt— sluggish; my joints were twingeing, especially my hips and knees. I want to be more energetic as I get older. I want to be healthy. —Jean, 61

What's your body mass index (BMI)?

Start by working out your BMI—the most common way of measuring whether or not someone is overweight. You need to take height into account because someone who is 168 lb (76 kg) and 5 ft (1.52 m) tall is overweight, whereas for someone who is around 6 ft (1.82 m), 168 lb is a healthy weight.

BMI is calculated as your weight divided by your height squared. So, for example, the average women in the UK weighs 157 lb (71.2 kg) and is 5 ft 4 in (1.62 m) tall, which means she has a BMI of 27.1—above the healthy range of 18.5–24.9. A BMI of 25–29.9 is classified as overweight, with increased health risks, and a BMI of 30 or more is classified as obese, with even greater health risks. The healthiest BMI is actually around 20–22. A BMI higher than this can start to increase your risk of cancer and other diseases. The higher your BMI, the greater your risk.

But BMI is only part of the story—two people can be the same height and weight but carry vastly different amounts of body fat. A woman with a BMI of 27 who does no exercise could have as much as 43 percent of her weight as fat, while another might be an athlete with lots of muscle and only 19 percent of her weight as fat. So while they both have a BMI that puts them in the overweight category, one has three times the amount of body fat and, as a result, very different health risks.

How to measure your body fat

If possible, try to measure your body fat, as this will give you the best indication of how overweight you are. You can buy yourself a set of stand-on scales or a handheld monitor that will measure your body fat for around $30 to $50, but you'll also find these available to use in some pharmacies and shopping centers. These machines work by passing a tiny, imperceptible

BODY MASS INDEX CALCULATOR

Body Weight (pounds)

Height (inches)	Normal						Overweight					Obese										Extreme Obesity														
BMI	19	20	21	22	23	24	25	26	27	28	29	30	31	32	33	34	35	36	37	38	39	40	41	42	43	44	45	46	47	48	49	50	51	52	53	54
58	91	96	100	105	110	115	119	124	129	134	138	143	148	153	158	162	167	172	177	181	186	191	196	201	205	210	215	220	224	229	234	239	244	248	253	258
59	94	99	104	109	114	119	124	128	133	138	143	148	153	158	163	168	173	178	183	188	193	198	203	208	212	217	222	227	232	237	242	247	252	257	262	267
60	97	102	107	112	118	123	128	133	138	143	148	153	158	163	168	174	179	184	189	194	199	204	209	215	220	225	230	235	240	245	250	255	261	266	271	276
61	100	106	111	116	122	127	132	137	143	148	153	158	164	169	174	180	185	190	195	201	206	211	217	222	227	232	238	243	248	254	259	264	269	275	280	285
62	104	109	115	120	126	131	136	142	147	153	158	164	169	175	180	186	191	196	202	207	213	218	224	229	235	240	246	251	256	262	267	273	278	284	289	295
63	107	113	118	124	130	135	141	146	152	158	163	169	175	180	186	191	197	203	208	214	220	225	231	237	242	248	254	259	265	270	278	282	287	293	299	304
64	110	116	122	128	134	140	145	151	157	163	169	174	180	186	192	197	204	209	215	221	227	232	238	244	250	256	262	267	273	279	285	291	296	302	308	314
65	114	120	126	132	138	144	150	156	162	168	174	180	186	192	198	204	210	216	222	228	234	240	246	252	258	264	270	276	282	288	294	300	306	312	318	324
66	118	124	130	136	142	148	155	161	167	173	179	186	192	198	204	210	216	223	229	235	241	247	253	260	266	272	278	284	291	297	303	309	315	322	328	334
67	121	127	134	140	146	153	159	166	172	178	185	191	198	204	211	217	223	230	236	242	249	255	261	268	274	280	287	293	299	306	312	319	325	331	338	344
68	125	131	138	144	151	158	164	171	177	184	190	197	203	210	216	223	230	236	243	249	256	262	269	276	282	289	295	302	308	315	322	328	335	341	348	354
69	128	135	142	149	155	162	169	176	182	189	196	203	209	216	223	230	236	243	250	257	263	270	277	284	291	297	304	311	318	324	331	338	345	351	358	365
70	132	139	146	153	160	167	174	181	188	195	202	209	216	222	229	236	243	250	257	264	271	278	285	292	299	306	313	320	327	334	341	348	355	362	369	376
71	136	143	150	157	165	172	179	186	193	200	208	215	222	229	236	243	250	257	265	272	279	286	293	301	308	315	322	329	338	343	351	358	365	372	379	386
72	140	147	154	162	169	177	184	191	199	206	213	221	228	235	242	250	258	265	272	279	287	294	302	309	316	324	331	338	346	353	361	368	375	383	390	397
73	144	151	159	166	174	182	189	197	204	212	219	227	235	242	250	257	265	272	280	288	295	302	310	318	325	333	340	348	355	363	371	378	386	393	401	408
74	148	155	163	171	179	186	194	202	210	218	225	233	241	249	256	264	272	280	287	295	303	311	319	326	334	342	350	358	365	373	381	389	396	404	412	420
75	152	160	168	176	184	192	200	208	216	224	232	240	248	256	264	272	279	287	295	303	311	319	327	335	343	351	359	367	375	383	391	399	407	415	423	431
76	156	164	172	180	189	197	205	213	221	230	238	246	254	263	271	279	287	295	304	312	320	328	336	344	353	361	369	377	385	394	402	410	418	426	435	443

Source: Adapted from Clinical Guidelines on the Identification, Evaluation, and Treatment of Overweight and Obesity in Adults: The Evidence Report.

electric current through your body. Your lean tissues (i.e., muscle and organs) contain mainly water and electrolytes that conduct this current, whereas fat, which contains little or no water, isn't a good conductor and impedes the current. By measuring how much lean tissue you have, the monitor estimates how much fat you have from your overall weight (i.e., total weight – lean weight = fat weight). Stand-on scales, which send a current through your lower body, are more accurate than handheld monitors, which just measure your arms, although stand-on scales are not foolproof. They will underestimate your fat levels if you have extra fluid in your body—for example, for women, around the time of your period—or if you have internal metalwork, such as metal joint replacements. They will also overestimate your fat level if you are dehydrated.

For best results, use a body fat monitor at the same time of day, once a week, ideally first thing in the morning. Wear minimal clothing, empty your bladder before use, and avoid using the device straight after exercising, drinking alcohol, or eating. Please note that you shouldn't use body fat meters if you have a pacemaker.

Alternatively, you can use our Body Fat Percentage Calculator (see Appendix A, page 313), which estimates your body fat from your weight, height, age, and sex.

As a general guide, women should have between 20 percent and 34 percent of their body weight as fat, and men should have between 8 percent and 25 percent.[1]

I had to do something—I was constantly worrying about my weight, I had no interest in clothes, and I was always planning a diet. Something had to change. —Sandra, 49

Check your waistline

For certain health risks—for example, heart disease and diabetes—your waist measurement may be even more important than your weight. Some people gain weight on their bottoms and thighs (making them classic "pear" shapes), while others pile it on around their waist (making them classic "apple" shapes). Men are typically more apple shaped than women, especially if they have "beer bellies," but as women get older, they tend to gain weight around their middles rather than their hips and thighs. Contrary to what many people think, this weight redistribution can start to happen before menopause.[2]

If you're an "apple" with extra fat around your middle, the odds are that you also have a lot of extra fat stored on the inside, around the vital organs inside your abdomen. This internal fat is very dangerous for your health, causing inflammation in the body, which in turn increases the risk of type 2 diabetes, heart disease, stroke, and possibly some cancers. This intra-abdominal fat can be seen clearly in the scans below.

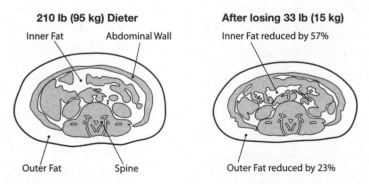

210 lb (95 kg) Dieter

Inner Fat   Abdominal Wall

Outer Fat   Spine

After losing 33 lb (15 kg)

Inner Fat reduced by 57%

Outer Fat reduced by 23%

These two scans were taken across the abdomen using magnetic resonance imaging. They were taken on the same person before and after losing 33 lb (15 kg). You can see that the right-hand scan after dieting is smaller than the left. The white areas are fat. You can see the fat as a layer under the skin and also in the abdomen. The gray areas are muscle and bone in the spine and the organs and bowels in the abdomen. This 40-year-old woman, who had a strong family history of breast cancer, lost 33 lb (15 kg) over the six months between the two scans. This represents about one-sixth (15.5 percent) of her overall body weight, and her BMI changed from 32 to 26.

In general, you have a higher risk of health problems if your waist is too large. As a guide, your waist should be less than half your height. Our research on 105,000 women found that women with a waist measurement of 36 in (90 cm) or more had a 40 percent greater risk of breast cancer, compared with women with a waist of 29 in (73 cm).[3] Use the chart below to check your waist measurement. It will help you to work out if you have too much inner fat and need to lose weight.

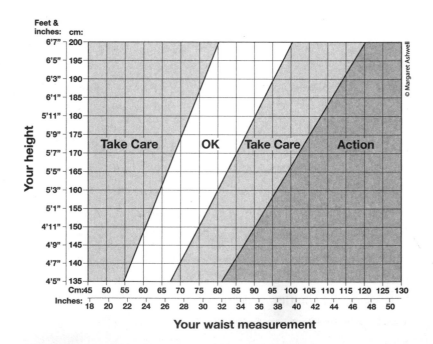

Your waist measurement

My joints ached when I woke up.
I was breathless if I had to run up a flight of stairs. I
couldn't fit into any of my clothes, my arms were wobbly,
I looked frumpy, old, and middle aged . . . shall I go on?
—Charlotte, 41

Commit to change

We know from the experiences of our Dieters that commitment is the key to making The 2-Day Diet work for you, even
if other diets have failed. Making changes to your diet and lifestyle isn't easy, but being committed, motivated, and prepared
for the challenge ahead is vital to your weight-loss success.

Why do you want to lose weight?

There may be lots of reasons—to improve your health, reduce
your chances of developing cancer, or have more energy for
playing with your children or grandchildren. For many of us
the big motivator is to look better, feel more confident, and
be able to wear nicer clothes. We often find that many dieters worry that this is self-indulgent and not a valid reason for
weight loss—and as a result they find it hard to admit that this
is their motivator. Whatever your motivation, it's important
that you are losing weight for yourself rather than to please or
placate someone else.

List your reasons for wanting to lose weight and the positive benefits you stand to achieve for your health, well-being,
and self-esteem. Then write "I am committed to losing weight
because . . ." and add your reasons. Put this somewhere where
you will see it every day—on your office wall, the fridge, or the
kitchen bulletin board. It will give you a daily reminder of why
you are doing the diet and will help you when you are having
a difficult day or feel like giving up.

I'm due to turn 50 this year, and I've dieted on and off for most of my adult life. I was just fed up with it all. I needed something that will last. —Vicky, 49

Is now the right time to diet?

Losing weight isn't just about willpower. It's hard to take on any new challenge if you're too stressed, have lots of other changes happening in your life, or haven't got the support of the people around you. Ask yourself:

▶ How are my stress levels—do I feel in control of my life?

▶ Do I have the support of my friends and family?

▶ Can I persuade any of my friends, colleagues, and/or family to do The 2-Day Diet with me for moral support and motivation? A bit of gentle competition can spur you on when you are dieting and keep you on track and focused on your goal.

▶ Am I confident that I will be able to make the changes to my diet?

▶ Can I see a way to plan meals and fit regular exercise into my daily life?

If you answer yes to most of these questions, you're probably ready to get going on The 2-Day Diet. If not, it's time to think about ways to manage your stress levels and find the support you will need to make The 2-Day Diet work for you.

Getting the support you need

If you've been on a diet before, you will know that there are plenty of diet saboteurs out there: the partner who wants you to stay "cuddly"; the friend who persuades you to eat that piece of cake "just this once"; or the mom who tells you that you were never designed to be thin. Having the wholehearted support of your nearest and dearest can really make a difference to your diet success, so it is important to bring people on board from day one. Watch out for sabotaging behavior—tempting you with forbidden foods, critical comments about how the Diet has "changed" you, suggestions that you're "not one of us" anymore. These are often difficult issues and may involve friends or family who are overweight themselves and don't like to see someone doing what they should be doing. Or they may be partners who feel threatened by seeing their other half gaining confidence and becoming more attractive to others. It is tempting to try to ignore such comments; however, we have found that when dieters clearly explain their reasons for trying to lose weight and actively ask for people's support, the sabotage stops and is replaced by support. One of our dieters described how taken aback she was by her work colleagues' negative response to her dieting. "They used to put chocolates and cookies on the table, and I was amazed by their response to me not wanting a cookie, so I actually stood up and said, look, cards on the table, and explained that I was dieting to reduce my risk of breast cancer. When I explained things, they were positive and supportive, but it took me doing that for them to really engage in it."

How do you feel about yourself?

Very few of us are totally happy with our size, shape, or how we look, especially when we are overweight. But for some people these negative feelings are so powerful that they have a major impact on their confidence, self-esteem, and the way they live their lives. It's crucial to acknowledge and address negative feelings before you start dieting, because if you feel bad about yourself, it can be even harder to make healthy lifestyle changes and lose weight.

If this sounds like you, give yourself time to stop and think carefully about how you see yourself and how your body image affects your day-to-day life and your ability to cope with new people or situations. It might take some time to think through the issues, but it will be time well spent and can only improve your chances of success. Try to focus on what you like about yourself as a person, the things you like about your appearance, and the positives about your life rather than dwelling on the things you want to change.

Manage your stress

Food and drink can become a refuge when life gets on top of you, so stress can be a major player in the struggle to control weight. The first step is to identify what causes stress in your life and to learn to recognize its telltale symptoms. You then need to find ways to reduce and manage your stress levels without resorting to food. The following steps may take a bit of time to consider, but it will be time well spent.

1. Make a list

List the main stresses in your life. They may include work issues, relationships, separation, family demands, bereavement, money problems, juggling too many roles, spreading yourself too thinly, the general pace of life, fear of failure, lack of support, feeling guilty about taking time and space for yourself, or practical things such as driving a car. Issues surrounding diet, weight, exercise, and health are often a source of concern and guilt.

2. Learn to recognize your stress symptoms

Common signs include feeling that you can't switch off, are not coping well, are not being efficient; feeling wound up, panicked, unable to support others; feeling you are letting people down. You may feel tired, develop headaches, feel tense and achy, have problems sleeping, or become irritable and anxious. You may find yourself eating more, or sometimes less, or drinking more alcohol than you usually do.

3. Develop your coping strategy

How you manage stress will depend on what works best for you. Review the list of stressful things in your life and take a long, hard look at how you can reduce the pressure on yourself. Put your stresses in order of priority, with the must-do's at the top. Starting at the bottom of the list, think about what you might be able to cross off or delegate to other people. If life feels out of control because of piles of unpaid bills or clutter everywhere, make a decision to tackle it, a little at a time. Getting organized can be a great antidote to stress. And if you're the kind of person who is always ready to step in when other people need help—and end up feeling overloaded as a result—start saying no. It will be hard at first, but the more often you do it, the easier it gets.

Find ways to make time for yourself. If you feel that you're running on empty, try to carve out some space in the week (ideally every day) to do whatever helps you to wind down. What we do to destress is very individual, and what works for you may not appeal to someone else. Some of the best ways to destress are also the simplest: get outside and walk—even a 10-minute walk, ideally in natural light, will help to recharge your batteries; join a choir—singing has been shown to help reduce stress and improve mood;[4] have a laugh—watch a funny film, read an amusing book, spend time with friends who make you laugh; book yourself a spa day, massage, or facial; go to a football game; catch up with friends who make you feel good (not the ones who make endless demands and sap your energy); turn up the volume and listen to your favorite music at full blast; invest in a relaxation tape or find a yoga or meditation class; make time for sex in your life.

Plan for success

As well as listing the benefits of losing weight, spend some time thinking about the challenges you might encounter along the way. If you've dieted before, you probably already have a good idea of the kind of problems that you are up against, whether it's losing motivation, giving in to temptation, or feeling unsupported by your nearest and dearest. By acknowledging and addressing these issues now, you will be ready to deal with the problems if and when they arise. Use a table like the one below to help you.

Benefits of doing The 2-Day Diet:	Problems I may encounter on The 2-Day Diet:
e.g., I will lose weight, feel better about myself, have more energy.	e.g., Other people may try to persuade me to break the diet; being tempted to snack in the evenings.
Benefits of not doing The 2-Day Diet:	Problems with not doing The 2-Day Diet:
e.g., Being able to eat whatever I want and whenever I want	e.g., I may gain more weight; I will feel more sluggish and have less energy.

Set your weight-loss goals

Your goal is to reach your ideal weight as quickly as possible, but, as every dieter knows, weight loss takes time. We know that good, rapid weight loss from day one boosts motivation and is a real incentive to carry on[5]—and the good news is that you can expect to see results quickly with The 2-Day Diet (see page 15). We found that our 2-Day Dieters not only lost weight about 50 percent more quickly than those on an every-day diet, but they were also able to change their eating patterns and reduce their appetite, which helped them to keep to the diet and maintain motivation.

It's good to have high ambitions, to aim to get back into a size 8 pair of jeans, or 32-inch-waist jeans for men, or to look good in a bathing suit. However, it pays to be realistic about how much weight you will lose and how long it will take to lose it. As you may recall, our 2-Day Dieters initially lost, on average, between 1 and 3 lb (0.5 and 1.4 kg) a week, which slowed down slightly so that by the end of three months they had lost, on average, 13 lb (5.8 kg), and some had lost far more. When it comes to weight loss, it's slow and steady that wins the race, and our 2-Day Dieters who stuck with The 2-Day Diet were the biggest winners and saw the biggest changes. So there's absolutely no reason why your weight-loss goal shouldn't be ambitious, especially if you're convinced that you can rise to the challenge and keep going. However, your goal also needs to be realistic and achievable.

In the short term
—the first three months

Lose 5–10 percent of your weight

It may not sound like much, and it's almost certainly far less than your overall goal, but if you can initially lose and keep off just 5–10 percent of your weight—that's 9–18 lb (4–8 kg) if you weigh 176 lb (80 kg)—you may well see instant health benefits and will be reducing your risk of type 2 diabetes by 60 percent,[6] as well as cutting your risk of heart disease by 70 percent.[7] Our work has also shown that this amount of weight loss cuts the risk of breast cancer by 25–40 percent.[8]

Some people will lose the weight faster than others. If you follow The 2-Day Diet correctly, most of the weight you lose will be fat, and, crucially, you should lose a substantial amount of the fat stored around your vital organs in the abdomen. This is important as this intra-abdominal fat potentially poses the biggest threat to your health. Research has shown that losing relatively small amounts of weight (10 percent) can help you lose 40 percent of the fat stored in your liver (which is particularly dangerous for your health).[9] Your liver is the HQ for your body's metabolism—it regulates the levels of circulating fat and sugars. Because a fatty liver doesn't work efficiently, you can have higher blood levels of sugar and fats, which in turn can lead to heart disease, diabetes, and cancers as well as permanent liver damage.

Your longer-term goal

Everyone is different, and it will be up to you to determine your personal weight-loss goal and how you set it. You might want to aim for your chosen ideal weight or want to get back to a weight that felt right for you in the past. Don't be scared to be ambitious, as long as your goal is realistic and achievable. Many of our 2-Day Dieters more than fulfilled their weight-loss ambitions. It may help to define small interim goals for two- or three-month blocks that you have a real chance of achieving. This will boost your confidence and your motivation to arrive at your destination goal.

Summary

▶ Do your groundwork. Calculate your Body Mass Index, measure your waist, and work out your body fat level before you start The 2-Day Diet—to help you know how much weight you need to lose.

▶ Be clear about your reasons for wanting to lose weight and make sure you have the right support to start on a diet to give yourself the best possible chance of success.

▶ Set yourself clear short-term and long-term weight-loss goals so that you know what you are aiming for.

▶ Don't forget! Even losing small amounts of weight can substantially improve your overall health and lower your risk of disease.

3

how to do the two restricted days

In this chapter we're going to explain how to do your two restricted days on The 2-Day Diet. We've designed this diet to reduce your appetite so that you are less likely to feel hungry; meet all your nutritional requirements so that you won't need to take supplements; and ensure that you lose as much fat as possible and preserve as much calorie-burning muscle as you can. If you are vegetarian, The 2-Day Diet will also work for you, since vegetarian choices of protein foods are just as, and possibly more, filling than meat.

> # Warning!
>
> Don't be tempted to devise your own two-day low-calorie diet. It will not only be harder to do because it will almost certainly leave you feeling hungry, but a "made-up" diet that isn't nutritionally balanced is unlikely to deliver the same health or weight-loss benefits as The 2-Day Diet.

The beauty of The 2-Day Diet is its simplicity and the fact it only has to be done on two days of the week, ideally consecutive: two restricted days are easy enough to fit into the busiest lifestyle. You don't have to count calories or go hungry. All you need to do is to stick to the recommended foods listed, making sure that you include the minimum recommended servings but that you don't exceed the maximum. By your using these simple rules to retrain your eating habits, The 2-Day Diet will help to put you back in control of what you eat and help you lose weight.

The 2-Day Diet

▶ For two days each week you are allowed foods that are high in protein, healthy fats, low-fat dairy foods, some vegetables, and fruit. There's no calorie counting to do; just use the calculators (see pages 328–335) to check the minimum and maximum number of servings of each type of food you can eat, which are stated for men and women.

▶ For two days your intake of carbohydrates is limited to around 50 g per day. This is because research shows that carbs make you hungry! With minimal carbs, your body quickly shifts from storing fat to burning it. It is the by-products of this fat burning, partly ketones and partly other by-products, that suppress your appetite.

▶ We recommend that you do your two restricted days back-to-back to get the full benefits of the Diet. Our research found that doing the two days together makes dieting easier and ensures that you actually get around to doing the second day. It may also have extra health benefits.

The diet has totally transformed my eating habits and I actually look forward to my two restricted days! —Kate, 27

How much can I eat?

We haven't imposed a strict calorie restriction on the two restricted days because we found that The 2-Day Diet is so satisfying that Dieters naturally restrict the amount they eat. We have given you a guide to the maximum number of servings of each type of food, to help reassure you that you aren't eating too much. Remember that these are *maximum* allowances, and you don't have to eat the maximum amount—most of our Dieters didn't. Dieters often worry that if they don't eat enough, they won't lose weight, but this is definitely not the case. However, it is important that you have enough protein and electrolytes on the two restricted days. For this reason we recommend that you have at least the minimum recommended amounts of protein foods and that you try to have your dairy, fruit, and vegetables, but beyond this, only eat as much as you need and listen to your body. If you're not hungry, eat less! You will find details on all the serving sizes in Appendix B on pages 315–320 at the back of the book.

I thought The 2-Day Diet was going to be hard, but it was
so much easier than I expected. The scope of foods is vast,
and you can vary your meals so you don't get bored with
what you are eating. —Kerry, 32

On each of your two restricted days of The 2-Day Diet you can consume:

▶ Protein foods (chicken, fish, eggs, lean meat): a maximum of 12 servings for women and 14 for men.

▶ Fats (canola oil, olive oil, nuts, or avocado): a maximum of 5 servings for women and 6 servings for men.

▶ Dairy: 3 servings.

▶ Fruit: 1 serving.

▶ Vegetables: 5 servings.

▶ At least 2 quarts of water, tea, coffee, or other sugar-free or low-calorie drinks.

If you wish, you can also include:

▶ Sugar-free chewing gum or licorice root (available from health food shops).

▶ Up to 10 sugar-free mints.

Protein foods

You can eat generous amounts of the following protein foods on your two restricted days of The 2-Day Diet:

▶ For women: a minimum of 4 servings and a maximum of 12 servings from the list below per day.

▶ For men: a minimum of 4 servings and a maximum of 14 servings from the list below per day.

You can have any number of protein servings in a meal, but make sure you keep within the maximum daily allowances.

Protein	1 serving equal to:
Fresh or smoked* white fish (e.g., flounder or cod)	2 oz (60 g) (two fish-finger-sized pieces)
Canned tuna in brine or spring water	1½ oz (45 g)
Oily fish (fresh or canned) in tomato sauce or oil (drained) (e.g., mackerel, sardines, salmon, trout, tuna; smoked salmon* or trout* or kippers*)	1 oz (30 g)
Seafood (e.g., shrimp, mussels, crab)	1½ oz (45 g)
Chicken, turkey, or duck (cooked without the skin)	1 oz (30 g) (a slice the size of a playing card)
Lean beef, pork, lamb, rabbit, venison, or organ meats (fat removed)	1 oz (30 g) per serving to a maximum of 1 lb 1 oz (500 g) per week for women and 1 lb 4 oz (600 g) per week for men (including the two restricted days and five unrestricted days of The 2-Day Diet)
Lean bacon*	1 grilled slice
Lean ham*	2 medium or 4 wafer-thin slices
Eggs	1 medium/large egg

*See Salt (page 55).

Protein	1 serving equal to:
Tofu	1¾ oz (50 g)

You can include only *one* of the following protein foods on *each* restricted day as they contain some carbohydrate. They count toward your daily protein allowance.

Protein	Maximum	Servings
Textured vegetable protein (TVP)	maximum 1 oz (30 g) per day	3
Soy and edamame beans	2 oz (60 g) per day	2
Low-fat hummus	maximum 1 tablespoon ½ oz (15 g) per day	1
Quorn	maximum 4 oz (115 g) per day	4

What you need to know about protein

Protein is a key part of your two restricted days on The 2-Day Diet as well as the rest of the week, because it is the most filling food you can eat. In fact, research suggests that our appetites are fundamentally controlled by our need for protein, and the body will keep telling you that you are hungry until you have eaten enough of it. If you eat a diet that's low in protein, you need to consume a lot of calories before you reach this point—which may be one reason why so many people overeat, especially dieters striving to keep to one of the numerous low-protein, low-fat weight-loss diet plans. Protein is also vital for maintaining muscle mass when you diet. Dieters who have successfully lost weight seem to be more likely to overeat and regain the weight they have lost if they have lost a lot of muscle as well as fat when they lost weight. This is a "feedback," which is the body's way of trying to replace the muscle lost through dieting. Protein foods are also helpful to dieters because they burn an extra 65–70 calories to absorb and digest them.

Fats

You can have generous amounts of the following foods:

▶ For women: a maximum of 5 servings from the list below per day.

▶ For men: a maximum of 6 servings per day.

Fat	1 serving equal to:
Margarine or low-fat spread (avoid the "buttery" types)	1 teaspoon (8 g)
Olive oil or other oil (not palm, coconut, or ghee)	2 teaspoons (7 g)
Oil-based dressing	2 teaspoons (7 g)
Unsalted or salted* or dry-roasted nuts (not honey roast)	2 teaspoons or 3 walnut halves, 3 Brazil nuts, 4 almonds, 8 peanuts, 10 cashews, or 10 pistachios (not chestnuts)
Pesto	1 teaspoon (8 g)
Mayonnaise	1 teaspoon (5 g)
Low-fat mayonnaise	1 tablespoon (15 g)
Olives*	10
Almond or cashew butter	1 teaspoon (8 g)

* See Salt (page 55).

You can have only one of the following fatty foods on each restricted day, as they contain some carbohydrate. They count toward your fat serving allowance.

Fat	Maximum	Servings
Avocado	½ pear	2
Guacamole	2 tablespoons	2
Low-fat guacamole	2 tablespoons	1

Dairy foods

Choose up to three servings from the following list per day:

Dairy	1 serving equal to:
Milk (1% or fat-free)	7 fl oz (200 ml)
Soy or almond milk (unsweetened with added calcium)*	7 fl oz (200 ml)
Yogurt: diet fruit, plain soy, or plain Greek (all low-fat)	4–5 oz (120–150 g) or 3 heaping tablespoons
Whole-milk plain yogurt	2½–3 oz (80–90 g) or 2 heaping tablespoons
Cottage cheese, low-fat	2½ oz (75 g) or 2 tablespoons
Low- or fat-free ricotta	3 oz (90 g) or 3 tablespoons
Cream cheese (light or extra-light)	1 oz (30 g) or 1 tablespoon
Lower-fat cheeses: low-fat cheddar, Edam, smoked Gouda, feta,† Camembert, ricotta, mozzarella, low-fat halloumi	Matchbox size: 1 oz (30 g) per serving, to a maximum of 4 oz (120 g) for women per week and 5 oz (150 g) for men on restricted and unrestricted days

* Don't be tempted to use rice or oat milk instead of dairy, soy, or almond milk. They are unsuitable for restricted days as they are too low in protein and too high in carbohydrates. However, you can use them on the five unrestricted days.

† See Salt (page 55).

Strangely for me, I didn't have cravings for chocolate or cookies on my two restricted days, but I did long for bread, cereals, and other not-so-naughty food experiences.

—Val, 43

Fruit

You can include one piece of fruit, but only the lower-carbohydrate fruits from the list below. If you prefer you can have an extra vegetable serving instead of fruit. You can sweeten fruit with artificial sweeteners, as required, but do not add sugar.

Fruit	1 serving equal to 80 g (2½ oz)
Apricots	3 fresh or dried
Blackberries	1 handful
Grapefruit	½ whole fruit
Melon	2 in (5 cm) slice
Papaya	1 slice
Peach	1 medium
Pineapple	1 large slice
Raspberries	2 handfuls
Strawberries	7
Stewed rhubarb or cranberries, with sweetener	3 heaping tablespoons

It was easier than I expected, and it's got easier as time has gone on. I soon got into the habit of eating less on the restricted days and have become used to eating less. I think it also helped to eat the same kind of food over the two days, making serving sizes easy to follow.—Lyndsey, 35

The 2-Day Diet makes me feel good because it gives me control and focus for two days of the week.—Carol, 39

Vegetables

Only the following lower-carbohydrate vegetables are allowed.
Choose five servings of vegetables per day from the list below.

Vegetables	1 serving equal to 2½ oz (80 g)
Artichoke	2 globe hearts
Asparagus, canned	7 spears
Asparagus, fresh	5 spears
Beans, broad	4 heaping tablespoons
Beans, string	4 heaping tablespoons
Bean sprouts, fresh	2 handfuls
Bell pepper (green only)	½
Bitter melon or summer squash	½
Broccoli	2 spears
Brussels sprouts	8
Cabbage	⅙ small cabbage or 3 heaping tablespoons shredded leaves
Cabbage, Chinese (napa)	⅕ head
Cauliflower	8 florets
Celeriac	3 heaped tablespoons
Celery	3 sticks
Corn, baby (whole, not kernels; available canned)	6
Cucumber	5 in (2 cm) piece
Dandelion greens, cooked	4 heaping tablespoons
Eggplant	⅓ medium
Fennel	½ cup sliced
Kale, curly, cooked	4 heaping tablespoons
Leeks	1 medium

Vegetables	1 serving equal to 2½ oz (80 g)
Lettuce (mixed leaves) or arugula	1 cereal bowlful
Mushrooms, fresh	14 buttons or 3 handfuls of slices
Mushrooms, dried	2 tablespoons or 1 handful porcini
Okra	16 medium
Pak choi	2 handfuls
Pumpkin	3 heaping tablespoons
Radishes	10
Scallions	8
Snow peas	1 handful
Spinach, cooked	2 heaping tablespoons
Spinach, fresh	1 cereal bowlful
Tomato, canned	2 plum tomatoes or ½ can chopped
Tomato, fresh	1 medium or 7 cherry
Tomato puree	1 heaping tablespoon
Tomato, sun-dried	4 pieces
Watercress	1 cereal bowlful
Zucchini	½ large

Flavorings

You can use these flavorings freely:

▶ Lemon juice

▶ Fresh or dried herbs and spices

▶ Black pepper

▶ Mustard/horseradish

▶ Vinegars—e.g., red or white wine vinegar, balsamic vinegar, or rice wine vinegar

▶ Fresh or prechopped garlic or ginger

▶ Chilies—fresh, powdered, or dried flakes

▶ Soy sauce/low-salt soy sauce (look for varieties with added chili for an extra kick!)*

▶ Miso paste

▶ Fish sauce*

▶ Worcestershire sauce*

Salt

Because you will be burning fat on your restricted days and losing water and electrolytes from your body, it's important to ensure that you take in some salt. You don't need huge amounts: include up to 5–6 g salt on those days (the equivalent of 2,000–2,400 mg sodium).

If you find that you are developing headaches on your restricted days, this may indicate that you need a little more salt.

There is some salt naturally occurring in some of the foods you will eat—for example, dairy foods, fish, and seafood. If you wish, you can include 4–6 servings of foods that are higher in salt on your restricted days. These foods are indicated in the food lists above with an asterisk (*).

Alternatively, you can include one of the following:

▶ ½ cube or 2 teaspoons bouillon as a drink or in food

▶ 1 tablespoon soy sauce

▶ 1 teaspoon yeast extract or meat stock with hot water

▶ 3 teaspoons gravy powder or granules dissolved in hot water

Do not include a salty drink or salty foods if you are taking a diuretic for high blood pressure.

Since too much salt is bad for blood pressure and bones, we recommend you limit these salty foods during the rest of the week to just one serving per week (see page 72).

> *I have found this diet really easy to follow. I can still eat a wide variety of foods and I love that I only need to wait a day or two if I have a serious chocolate or cake craving. Even better, I don't feel guilty about it when I do treat myself. I plan my two diet days around my social life, so it doesn't interfere at all. I plan my two days carefully to eat foods that will sustain me and keep me going, while giving me the nutrients I need. I do feel healthier and lighter on my toes!*
> —Andrea, 30

Ideas for low-calorie drinks

It is very important to drink plenty on your two restricted days of The 2-Day Diet. Aim to drink 2 quarts from the following list to prevent dehydration, constipation, and headaches, and to help keep hunger pangs at bay:

▶ Water (still or sparkling).

▶ Tea and coffee (black or add milk as required from your daily milk allowance; use sweeteners as required).

▶ Flavored sugar-free sparkling water—make sure you check the label and avoid brands containing added sugar.

▶ Sugar-free or no-added-sugar fruit-flavored drinks made with still or sparkling water. Avoid high-juice varieties, because they contain natural fruit sugars; instead, choose no-added-sugar varieties sweetened with artificial sweeteners.

▶ Fruit, herbal, or green teas.

▶ Diet, sugar-free, or no-added-sugar carbonated drinks (up to 3 quarts per week—see page 86).

▶ Grated ginger in boiling water (and sweeteners as required). Drink hot or allow to cool first, then chill.

▶ Slice of lemon or lime in boiling water.

You can sweeten all drinks with artificial sweeteners as required. Do not add sugar (see page 73). See pages 243–244 for some refreshing drinks you can make.

The vegetarian 2-Day Diet

If you are vegetarian, you can easily follow The 2-Day Diet. The vegetarian version is similar, but as some vegetarian sources of protein contain carbohydrates, you will need to eat slightly less of the dairy foods since these also contain carbohydrates. Your selection of protein foods is more limited than for meat and fish eaters, but it is extremely important to include the recommended amounts of protein and low-fat dairy foods to make sure you don't get hungry. The recipe chapter for the two restricted days (see page 179) is packed with many interesting meals you can prepare with eggs, tofu, soybeans, and textured vegetable protein (TVP).

Protein foods

▶ For women: a minimum of 4 servings and a maximum of 12 servings from the following list per day.

▶ For men: a minimum of 4 servings and a maximum of 14 servings from the following list per day.

On your two restricted days of The 2-Day Diet you can have generous amounts of eggs and tofu within your daily allowance:

Protein	1 serving equal to:
Eggs	1 medium/large egg
Tofu	1¾ oz (50 g)

You can also choose up to six protein servings from the following list each day. Make sure that you get no more than 15 g per day of total carbohydrates from this section.

Protein	1 serving equal to:
Vegetarian sausage/burger with < 5 g carb	½
Textured vegetable protein, uncooked	2 teaspoons (⅓ oz/10 g)
Soybeans (frozen or cooked)	2 tablespoons (1 oz/30 g)
Low-fat hummus	1 tablespoon 1 oz (15 g)
Tempeh	1½ oz (40 g)
Quorn, ground or fillet	1 oz (30 g)
Edamame beans (frozen or cooked)	2 tablespoons (1 oz/30 g)

Note: Avoid burgers and fillets with a breadcrumb coating, as these will be higher in carbohydrates.

A word about eggs

Eggs have had a bad press, but contrary to popular belief, they are a great diet food that you can eat freely. They're high in protein, low in fat, contain only 70 calories a serving, and are a great source of vitamins A and D (an egg can provide 10 percent of your daily requirement of vitamin D), selenium, calcium, iron, zinc, and folate.

Although many people worry that eggs are high in cholesterol, they are not linked to heart disease, and a recent study found that people on a low-fat diet who ate two eggs each day lost weight, with no adverse effects on their cholesterol levels. In fact, their levels of the beneficial form of cholesterol in the body, the HDL cholesterol, actually increased.[1]

Dairy foods

You can have up to 2 oz (60 g) of lower-fat cheese, but no more than 4 oz (120 g) per week for women and 5 oz (150 g) for men, including the two restricted and five unrestricted days, such as:

▶ Low-fat cheddar

▶ Low-fat feta

▶ Low-fat mozzarella

▶ Low-fat smoked Gouda

▶ Low-fat Camembert

▶ Low-fat Edam

▶ Low-fat ricotta

▶ Low-fat halloumi

You can also choose two servings from the following list per day:

Dairy	1 serving equal to:
Milk (1% or fat-free)	7 fl oz (200 ml)
Soy or almond milk (unsweetened with added calcium)*	7 fl oz (200 ml)

Dairy	1 serving equal to:
Yogurt: diet fruit, plain soy, or plain Greek (all low-fat)	4–5 oz (120–150 g) or plain or 3 heaping tablespoons
Whole-milk plain yogurt	2½–3 oz (80–90 g) or 2 heaping tablespoons
Cottage cheese, low-fat	2½ oz (75 g) or 2 tablespoons
Cream cheese (light or extra-light)	1 oz (30 g) or 1 tablespoon

* Don't be tempted to use rice milk instead of dairy, soy, or almond milk. It is unsuitable for restricted days as it is too low in protein and too high in carbohydrates. However, you can use it on the five unrestricted days.

Make sure that you include the allowance of fat, vegetables, and fruit on your restricted days (see pages 50–57).

Your questions answered

Do I need to take a vitamin supplement on the two restricted days of The 2-Day Diet?

You don't need to take a supplement on The 2-Day Diet. When you go on any weight-loss diet and eat less, you often reduce your intake of vitamins and minerals. It's always better to get the nutrients you need from food, as this ensures a gradual supply of nutrients that are more easily absorbed by your body. The one-shot dose delivered in a supplement can lead to a flood of abnormally high levels, which may not be good for your body. For example, there is currently a concern that high-dose calcium supplements cause high blood levels of calcium, which can lead to calcification and damage to the arteries and possibly heart disease. The 2-Day Diet is designed to ensure that you get the nutrients you need. The nutrients that your diet may be lacking on the two restricted days of The 2-Day Diet are calcium, iron, zinc, and magnesium, and we find that many people, including our Dieters, will already have low intakes of selenium, folate, and vitamin A in their normal diet. Good sources of these important nutrients on your restricted days are:

▶ Calcium from low-fat dairy foods, calcium-fortified soy or almond milk, canned oily fish if you eat the bones, tofu set with calcium, almonds, eggs, and green leafy vegetables.

▶ Iron from lean meat, eggs, nuts, and green vegetables.

▶ Zinc from lean meat, milk, eggs, nuts, and cheese.

▶ Magnesium from lean meat, poultry, fish, Quorn, nuts, soy-beans, and green vegetables.

▶ Selenium from meat, fish, Brazil nuts, and eggs.

▶ Folate from asparagus and green leafy vegetables.

▶ Vitamin A from eggs, cheese, and margarines.

It is also important to include good dietary sources of these foods on unrestricted days too.

Should I be eating lots of nuts—aren't they very high in calories?

Many of our 2-Day Dieters worry about eating nuts because they are high in fat and therefore calories. However, they are packed with healthy monounsaturated and omega-3 fats (see page 76), and because they are high in protein, they are also very filling. They may even help reduce the risk of heart disease because they contain arginine, a substance that may make your artery walls more flexible and less prone to blood clots. Eat unsalted varieties of nuts to keep your salt intake down, unless you are using them as a salty food on the restricted days of The 2-Day Diet (see page 55).

How easy is The 2-Day Diet to follow?

Many of our 2-Day Dieters were surprised by how easy they found The 2-Day Diet. Because it is simple but structured, they quickly adapted to it and got into a routine. Only 3 percent of our 2-Day Dieters reported having problems fitting it into their daily lives and with family meals. You will need to plan ahead, but because you are dieting only for two days, making larger quantities and freezing them will give you a good range of different meals to choose from. Many of our 2-Day Dieters found that the 2-Day Diet actually became easier the longer they were on it. As one woman said, "Unlike other diets, which are okay at first and get harder over time, I found The 2-Day Diet quite hard to begin with, but it got easier the more your body and mind got used to what you were doing."

Will I be hungry on my diet days?

You should not feel any hungrier on your two restricted days of The 2-Day Diet than you do normally. We assessed "hungriness" in our 2-Day Dieters before starting the Diet and while they were doing it, using hunger scales. We found that they scored their hungriness exactly the same on their restricted and unrestricted days as they had before they started The 2-Day Diet. It can be easy to mistake hunger for thirst, so if you feel hungry, try having a drink and see if that helps. On the two restricted days of The 2-Day Diet, make sure that you have enough protein foods, nuts, dairy foods, and vegetables, which are particularly good at filling you up. If you do feel hungry the first few times you try the Diet, stick with it, as most of our 2-Day Dieters found that it got easier as they got used to it.

Snack ideas for the two restricted days of The 2-Day Diet

- Olives.
- Handful of nuts (not chestnuts).
- Fruit from the allowed list.
- Vegetable crudités, such as celery, cucumber, green peppers, snow peas, scallions, and cherry tomatoes, with salsa, low-fat hummus, tuna pâté, tzatziki, or guacamole (see pages 193–196).
- Plain or diet yogurt.
- Bowl of soup (see page 186).
- Salad or cooked vegetables with low-fat cottage cheese, low-fat cream cheese, or hummus.
- ½ cup of low-fat cottage cheese.
- Smoothie made with yogurt, fat-free or 1% milk, and one piece of fruit.
- Half a can of sardines.
- Salty drink (see page 55).
- Sautéed tofu or chicken strips lightly fried in spices.
- Boiled egg.
- Avocado, mozzarella, tomato, and basil skewers or stacks.
- Celery sticks filled with low-fat cream cheese.
- Asparagus spears dipped in soft-boiled egg.
- Sugar-free Jell-O.
- Popsicle made from frozen, diluted fruit-flavored drink.

Will The 2-Day Diet help me to permanently change my eating habits?

The two restricted days of The 2-Day Diet helped our Dieters recognize their habitual "unhealthy" eating habits and behaviors. The two restricted days helped them to practice and get into the habit of eating healthier foods and smaller servings each week. On top of that, they began to recognize, often for the first time in a long time, what was "real" hunger or thirst, rather than just wanting to eat for the sake of it. They learned to really enjoy and savor their food both on the two restricted days and on the five unrestricted days. The 2-Day Diet helps put you back in control of your eating.

Why am I urinating more?

One thing you will notice on your restricted days is that you will be going to the bathroom more often. This is for two reasons: First, because you will be mobilizing glycogen, the carbohydrate stored in your muscles and liver; this releases water into the body that the body then needs to get rid of. Second, burning fat also increases the levels of ketones in the blood; this acts as a diuretic (in the same way as tea and coffee), making you want to urinate more.

Ketones are a natural by-product of burning fat in the body. They are not thought to have harmful effects unless they build up to extremely high levels, which won't happen on The 2-Day Diet. Ketones have a bad press, as the levels achieved with some daily very low-carbohydrate diets can lead to side effects such as headaches, nausea, or bad breath. Our Dieters typically doubled their level of ketones, in contrast to dieters on longer-term low-carbohydrate diets, who experience five-fold increases in ketones.

Will I feel more tired on my diet days?

Quite the contrary! Most of our 2-Day Dieters were very positive about the way they felt while doing the Diet. Many said they felt invigorated, cleansed, and detoxed during and after the two restricted days each week. This made them more committed and more motivated to keep to The 2-Day Diet each week and, importantly, to eat healthily for the rest of the week. They reported feeling less bloated after eating, less sluggish, and more energetic, and when we assessed their general mood and well-being, we found that their scores for tension, depression, anger, fatigue, and confusion were halved, while in nearly all cases their mood improved.

Interestingly, our 2-Day Dieters said that the two restricted days each week gave them all the positive feelings that dieters often experience during the first few days of following a normal diet, with the positive feelings of increased energy and sense of achievement that go with it. Revisiting those feelings every week gave them a real boost and reinforced their motivation to succeed.

Are there any side effects?

None of our 2-Day Dieters reported major problems, although a few experienced headaches. If this happens, make sure you are drinking plenty (2 quarts a day is usually enough). You can drink more than this, but you will need to ensure you are including enough electrolytes as well—i.e., potassium, sodium (salt), and also magnesium—which you will get by eating your recommended servings of fruit, vegetables, dairy, and protein foods. You may find you need to include a salty food or drink on the two restricted days of The 2-Day Diet (see page 55). Although it's not necessary to cut down on tea and coffee on the Diet, if you find you are drinking less of these than usual since starting it, your headaches may be related to caffeine withdrawal. The drop in carbohydrate intake on the two days can also cause headaches, but this should improve as your body gets used to it.

A few 2-Day Dieters found they became constipated. If this happens, make sure you are getting enough fluid and having your full fruit and vegetable allowance on restricted days. On your unrestricted days, make sure you eat plenty of fiber by having your full allowance of fruit and vegetables, choosing carbohydrates that are high in fiber (see page 336), drinking plenty, and meeting the recommendations for exercise.

I'm worried that I won't be able to concentrate at work on my restricted days

A few Dieters—again only 3 percent—found concentration difficult, although it is possible that they were expecting problems and so any effects were exaggerated. There's no consistent evidence that either low-calorie or low-carbohydrate diets affect concentration. In one recent study in the USA, students were given either a very low-calorie drink (150 cal, 30 g carbohydrates) or a drink that contained their full calorie requirement (2,300 cal, 560 g carbohydrate) per day for two days without being told which drink they were getting. None receiving the low-calorie drink reported any problems with concentration, energy levels, or mood.[2] Other research suggests that low-carb, high-protein diets could actually increase memory and alertness[3] and have been used to treat older adults with cognitive impairment.[4]

If you genuinely feel that you are struggling to concentrate or feel lightheaded:

▶ Make sure you are well hydrated and are getting enough salt (sodium, see page 55), potassium, and magnesium by including recommended foods.

▶ Make sure that you are getting the 50 g of carbohydrates allowed on restricted days (found in your dairy and fruit and vegetable allowances—see pages 51–54).

Will my breath smell on The 2-Day Diet?

A few of our Dieters complained about having a bad taste in their mouth, but this was usually minor and not enough to make their breath smell. The taste is caused by ketones, substances that build up when your body burns fat to use for energy. Although you may notice it on the two restricted days, it will disappear on the five unrestricted days. Drinking more may help, and you can also suck sugar-free mints (up to 10 a day).

Aren't the two days of The 2-Day Diet just the same as an Atkins- or Dukan-style diet?

The two restricted days of The 2-Day Diet are low-carb and so have some similarities to low-carb, high-protein diets such as Atkins or Dukan, but this diet is different. The low-carb days of The 2-Day Diet are designed for weight loss and are also designed for optimum health, ensuring that you get the right balance of healthy fats (low in saturates, high in monounsaturates and omega-3 fats) and fruit and vegetables. Remember, you are only eating low-carb for two days of the week. When you combine the two days with a healthy balanced Mediterranean diet for the rest of the week, it makes The 2-Day Diet very different from other diets.

How much will the diet cost—will my food bill go up?

The 2-Day Diet should cost you less than you are spending now. Before they started dieting, our Dieters spent, on average, $63 on food and drink for themselves each week. This included $54 on food and nearly $9 on alcohol. Of the money spent on food, nearly $9 was spent on frozen meals, $7 on takeout, and an average of $5 on sweets, cakes, and biscuits. On The 2-Day Diet, their total food bill dropped by $13 per week. They were now spending $50 a week on food and drink because they had cut back on frozen meals, alcohol, and sweet foods. You can either pocket the difference or set it aside to treat yourself when you reach your diet goals. One important change was that the amount they spent per calorie did increase with the higher nutritional quality of their diet—this rose from just under 3¢ per calorie to 4¢ per calorie. However, because they were eating fewer calories, their overall food bill was lower. The recipes and meal ideas in this book (see pages 169–311) include plenty of healthy and reasonably priced options, so being on The 2-Day Diet does not mean that you have to spend more on food.

Summary

▶ For the two restricted days of The 2-Day Diet, you are limited to eating protein, fats, five servings of low-carb vegetables, one serving of fruit, and some low-fat dairy foods. It's important to stick to the restricted foods, to not exceed the maximum number of servings allowed, and to get enough protein, which will help to keep you full and maintain muscle in your body.

▶ No high-carbohydrate foods such as bread, cake, sweets, or alcohol are allowed on the two restricted days.

▶ You don't need to take any supplements, as The 2-Day Diet is balanced to meet all your nutritional needs.

▶ To get the full benefits of the Diet, do your two restricted days together (one after the other).

▶ The majority of Dieters find the two restricted days of The 2-Day Diet are easy to adapt to and to fit into their lifestyle.

▶ Most Dieters don't feel hungry. Instead they feel healthier and have more energy while doing the Diet. A small minority may experience minor side effects, which are easily remedied.

4

how to eat
on the five
unrestricted days

Your diet for the remaining days (the five unrestricted days) on The 2-Day Diet should be based on eating a healthy Mediterranean-style diet. This includes food that is as whole and unprocessed as possible, with lots of fruit and vegetables, whole grains, beans, nuts, and olive oil, as well as fish, poultry, and low-fat dairy foods. It can include small amounts of lean red meat—but not lots of pasta, pizza, and red wine!

The Mediterranean diet

The Mediterranean diet is packed full of disease-fighting anti-oxidants, vitamins, and flavonoids, and the benefits of eating this way are almost too numerous to list. There's convincing evidence that it not only lowers the risk of heart disease and type 2 diabetes but may also protect against some cancers and Alzheimer's disease.[1] Your eating plan for these five unrestricted days contains high-protein, high-fiber foods to help you feel full and reduce your chances of overeating. Don't be tempted to overeat or eat junk food on these five unrestricted days—follow the guidelines below to give yourself the best possible chance of successful weight loss. A full guide to recommended servings for the unrestricted days can be found in Appendix C (see pages 321–326).

Protein foods
Include:
▶ White or oily fish and seafood.

▶ Chicken, turkey, or duck (cooked without skin).

▶ Lean cuts of red meat—for example, beef, pork, lamb, or organ meats—lean game, venison, rabbit, or pheasant (maximum 1 lb 1 oz/500 g a week for women and 1 lb 4 oz/600 g a week for men, including the two restricted and five unrestricted days of The 2-Day Diet).

▶ Beans, chickpeas, and lentils—use these for bulking up dishes.

Limit to once during the five unrestricted days
▶ Fatty cuts of red meat, poultry, and game (these are high in saturated fat).

▶ High-fat processed meat and meat products (for example, sausage and corned beef—these are high in saturated fat and salt).

▶ Charred and well-done meat and fish (these are limited

because of concerns about cancer risk associated with consuming charred foods).

▶ Battered/breaded fish (these are higher in calories and much lower in protein than uncoated fish).

▶ Low-fat processed meats, bacon, ham, and salty fish such as kippers, smoked salmon, smoked mackerel, and smoked white fish—to limit your overall salt intake for the week.

You can include salty foods on your two restricted days as you may be losing fluid and salt from the body (see page 55).

All about carbs

Carbohydrates provide most of our energy—typically 50 to 60 percent of our calories. Contrary to popular belief, a traditional Mediterranean diet is not based on foods such as pasta and pizza but actually contains less than 45 percent of its calories as carbohydrates. Because your two restricted days contain very few carbohydrates, your overall 2-Day Diet for the week has around 40 percent of its energy from carbohydrates—more in line with our hunter-gatherer ancestors, who are thought to have obtained between 20 and 40 percent of their calories from carbohydrates.

When it comes to carbohydrates, choose whole-grain varieties whenever possible. They contain more fiber and nutrients than processed or white versions, take longer to digest and absorb, and can keep you feeling full for longer. Cut down on white, refined carbohydrates and sugar, and try to avoid sugary snacks such as sweets and cakes. These carbohydrates are quickly digested and lead to spikes in blood sugar and high levels of insulin, which in turn increase your appetite and leave you craving more!

Sugar provides four calories per gram but has no other nutrients, which is why it is often referred to as having "empty" calories. Too much of any kind of sugar is bad for you, but be particularly wary of foods containing added fructose (often labeled as "high-fructose corn syrup") found in some breakfast cereals, cereal bars, sweetened fruit juices or high-juice fruit drinks, yogurt, rice pudding, cookies, cakes, and ice cream.

There is growing concern about the damaging effects of fructose, both because of its high-calorie content and because it is directly converted to fat that builds up in the liver. A fatty liver is less able to remove fat circulating in the blood (see page 42) so this fat is deposited in the blood vessels, leading to narrowing of the vessels and raised blood pressure. In a recent study, people who ate an extra 1,000 calories in sweets and sugary drinks for three weeks showed an alarming threefold increase in the amount of fat in their livers. This was reversed when they subsequently followed a low-calorie Mediterranean diet.[2]

Fructose is also found naturally in fruit in far smaller amounts than in processed foods: an apple, for example, only contains one-fifth of the fructose of a regular can of cola. Fructose in fruit does not seem to have any adverse effects on health, as fruit also contains protective plant polyphenols. One of the reasons for the harmful effects of the modern Western diet is the large amounts of refined carbohydrates listed in the left-hand column of the table on page 74.

Switch from these carbs . . .	. . . to these
White bread, baguettes, bagels, croissants, crumpets	Pita bread, pumpernickel bread, multigrain bread, rye bread, whole wheat bread
White rice, white couscous, white noodles	Basmati rice, bulgur wheat, quinoa, brown rice, brown noodles, whole wheat pasta, brown couscous, brown rice
Cornflakes, white rice cereal, sugary cereals, instant oatmeal	Oatmeal, bran flakes, high-fiber bran cereal, shredded wheat, no-added-sugar muesli
Potato chips, sweets, cookies, sugary popcorn, doughnuts, cakes	Yogurt, nuts, plain popcorn
Mashed potatoes, French fries	Sweet potatoes, new potatoes boiled in their skins, baked potatoes
Plain crackers, rice cakes	Whole grain crackers, rye crispbreads
Sugary carbonated drinks	Water, sugar-free fruit drinks, carbonated diet drinks

The diet is easy as long as you are organized.
I haven't felt the need for chocolate, potato chips, etc.
This is dieting without feeling hungry and losing weight
without feeling deprived. —Chris, 63

Your "five a day"

We need fruit and vegetables to protect us from heart disease and strokes, to help control blood pressure, and to keep our bones healthy. Fruit and vegetables may also help protect against certain cancers, although the links with cancer are not as strong or compelling as they are for heart disease.[3] Fruit and vegetables may also reduce the risk of dementia.

On the two restricted days of The 2-Day Diet you are allowed to have five servings of lower-carbohydrate vegetables and one low-carbohydrate fruit, but for the five unrestricted days of the rest of the week you can include a variety of fruits and vegetables (including higher-carbohydrate ones). You should aim to have two servings of fruit and five servings of vegetables per day. Don't assume that eating fruit and vegetables will mean that you will naturally want to eat less of other foods. In fact, when researchers asked overweight people to include six to eight servings of fruit and vegetables a day in their diet, many just added this to what they normally ate and gained 4½ lb (2 kg) over the eight weeks of the study.[4]

We recommend eating more vegetables than fruit, as they usually provide fewer calories—for example a banana can contain between 80 and 160 calories, depending on size, while 20 mushrooms contain only 16 calories and a large serving of broccoli only 12 calories. Vegetables are a great way to fill up your plate while adding very few calories. As a dieter, you may already know that a small bar of chocolate provides 300 calories. For the same number of calories you could eat a whopping 19 lb (9 kg) of broccoli!

> *It's so great to be losing weight and knowing that I'm eating healthily. I love the fish, chicken, and salads on the Mediterranean days.* —Anna, 43

Fat facts

We all need some fat in our diet, but too much leads to us piling on the pounds (a gram of carbohydrate contains four calories, whereas a gram of fat contains nine). Therefore, try not to add extra fat when you are cooking, and opt for broiling, microwaving, or steaming when you can, and if you do use oil, just use a little olive, soy, or canola oil or a little cooking spray.

Cut down on saturated fats, since these are the harmful

fats that clog arteries. Saturated fats are found in fatty red meat, processed meats and sausages, full-fat dairy products, palm oil, chocolate, and coconut oil. Try to replace them with "healthy" fats, especially monounsaturated fats in olives, olive oil, canola oil, avocados, nuts (such as peanuts, almonds, pecans, hazelnuts, cashews, and pistachios), which can help to lower cholesterol levels.

Omega-3 fats have important roles for health, as they help to maintain a healthy heart and lower blood pressure and blood fat levels. They also have anti-inflammatory effects, which help to maintain a healthy brain and nervous system and reduce the risk of diabetes and certain cancers. The body also needs omega-6 fats; however, the modern diet contains too few omega-3 fats and an excess of omega-6s, which results in omega-3 fats not being able to carry out their good work.

The best way to redress the balance is to consume more omega-3s, found in oily fish such as salmon, sardines, mackerel, and fresh tuna (not canned) and, for vegetarians, omega-3-enriched eggs, flaxseed, walnuts, and canola oil. Don't overdo omega-6-rich foods such as corn, sunflower oil, turkey, game, shellfish, canned tuna, pine nuts, and sesame seeds.

I've always found diets difficult before—as life tends to get in the way. The 2-Day Diet's been so much easier, as you can work it around whatever else is going on. You can go to parties, weddings, and meals out and still lose weight!
—Mary, 31

Make sure you drink enough

Most of us don't drink anywhere near enough, and it's especially important to stay well hydrated when you are trying to lose weight. We recommend at least eight glasses of fluid each day

(2 quarts) to help you feel full, to keep you hydrated, and to prevent constipation. We often mistake thirst for hunger, so if you fancy something to eat, have a drink first and see if your cravings go away. In fact, some research suggests that drinking water before you eat could help you eat less at mealtimes—and drinking cold water may actually boost your metabolic rate for up to an hour after drinking.[5] However, don't get too excited! It will only burn five extra calories a day, but this can add up over the year—and every little bit helps. Some people worry about drinking too much, and there have been occasional reports of excessive water intake (more than 5 quarts per day) leading to water toxicity, with dilution of the salts in the blood. This is only really a problem if large volumes of water are drunk over a short time; you should ideally drink no more than 1 quart over an hour.

Normal nondiet carbonated drinks are a major problem in our Western diet. They are packed with sugar (about 10 teaspoons per can), contain around 150 calories, but contain no nutrients and are quickly converted to fat in the body.

What to drink

You need to drink at least 2 quarts from the following list a day:

▶ Water (still or sparkling).

▶ Tea—black or green, caffeinated or decaffeinated.

▶ Coffee—caffeinated or decaffeinated.

▶ Herbal and fruit teas.

▶ Sugar-free or diet fruit-flavored drinks or carbonated drinks (less than 3 quarts per week—see page 86).

Limit the following

▶ Alcohol.

▶ Adding sugar to drinks.

▶ Nondiet carbonated drinks.

▶ Fruit juice (a maximum of 7 fl oz/200 ml per day).

▶ Vegetable juice (a maximum of 7 fl oz/200 ml per day).

Fruit juice

People assume that a glass of pure, unsweetened fruit juice is a healthy addition to your meal. By all means have a glass a day, but it's always better to eat a piece of whole fruit instead. Not only is fruit juice high in calories, it contains no fiber and won't be as filling as eating a piece of fruit. In one study, people were given either an apple or some apple juice and were then asked to eat a meal until they were full. The apple eaters ate less at the meal and 15 percent fewer calories overall than those given juice to drink.[6]

Why fiber is important for your health and weight

Fiber is found in the plant foods we eat and is vital for anyone who is trying to lose weight and follow The 2-Day Diet. Fiber helps you feel full longer, keeps your blood sugar stable, and keeps your bowels functioning optimally. There are two main types of fiber, both of which are important for the Dieter.

Insoluble fiber

This is found in cereals and beans. It protects against constipation and helps keep your bowels healthy by preventing the buildup of toxic substances (the by-products of digested protein), which have been linked to bowel cancer. Since The 2-Day Diet includes plenty of protein, it is really important to make sure you have enough of this type of fiber on unrestricted days.

Soluble fiber

Found in oats, barley, beans, fruit, and vegetables, soluble fiber slows down the rate at which food empties from your stomach.

Why fiber is vital for your health

Fiber plays a key role in maintaining the balance of beneficial bacteria in your intestines. Each of us has about 100 trillion bacteria in our bowels (weighing around 4 lb/1.8 kg). Their number gives an indication of their importance to our health. Recent studies indicate that there are healthy combinations of bacteria, which if disrupted by poor diet can actually lead to diseases and even obesity. Bacteria ferment the fiber we eat and produce fats known as "short-chain" fats. Research indicates that eating plenty of fiber results in the right bacteria in the bowels, which then produce the right fats. These have three key roles in protecting our health:

- The fats are an essential fuel for the cells lining the bowels and keep these cells healthy.
- Some of the fats produced in the bowels are absorbed, circulate in the bloodstream, and reduce sugar levels and the levels of disease-producing fats in the blood.
- Having the right bacteria in the intestines may also affect your weight. Overweight people have a different balance of intestinal bacteria, which can cause weight gain.[7]

It also slows down the absorption of nutrients, avoiding surges in blood sugar after meals and helping to keep blood sugar stable. Soluble fiber helps to lower cholesterol too.

Make sure you include your permitted fruit and vegetables on the two restricted days of The 2-Day Diet. Aim to have at least 24 g of fiber a day on your unrestricted days, with a good mix of soluble and insoluble types (see Appendix E, page 336). Note that you will not be able to manage 24 g of fiber on the two restricted days and typically will manage around 14 g. If you are not used to fiber in your diet, it is best to increase your fiber intake gradually over two or three weeks—eating more fiber will inevitably create more gas, and consuming too much fiber too quickly can lead to bloating, discomfort, and flatulence. Make sure you drink more fluids when you increase your fiber intake—at least eight glasses of water or other low-calorie drinks daily.

Dairy foods

Like eggs, dairy foods have had a bad press in recent years. The claims that dairy foods can cause breast cancer have led many women to stop eating them, although despite extensive research, there is no evidence of a causal link. And for dieters, low-fat dairy foods are a positive asset. Milk protein seems to be particularly filling, and there's evidence that the calcium in dairy foods acts almost like a detergent, grabbing fat before it can be absorbed—it's only a small effect, but it probably amounts to around 45 calories a day that you don't have to lose elsewhere in your diet. The calcium in dairy foods may also benefit blood pressure and is vital for bone health. We've ensured that The 2-Day Diet is high in protein, calcium, vitamin D, and fruit and vegetables, which all help maintain healthy bones. This is important, since there is an inevitable small reduction in bone density when you diet, as you are lighter and your bones are carrying less weight. Don't forget that weight-bearing exercise is also an essential part of keeping bones strong (see page 123).

Aim to have at least 800 mg of calcium a day—that's the equivalent of 7 fl oz (200 ml) of milk, one yogurt, or half a can of salmon, provided you eat the bones too. If you don't enjoy, or are intolerant of, dairy products, make sure that you are getting plenty of calcium elsewhere in your diet (see below).

Calcium Calculator

Food	Calcium (mg)
Sardines (canned), if you eat the bones (3½ oz /100 g)	500
Mackerel (canned), if you eat the bones (3½ oz/100 g)	250
Salmon (canned), if you eat the bones (3½ oz/100 g)	300
Low-fat cheese such as Edam or low-fat cheddar (1 oz/30 g)	240
Soy, rice, almond (calcium fortified) (7 fl oz/200 ml)	240
Fruit juice with added calcium (7 fl oz/200 ml)	240
1% or fat-free milk (7 fl oz/200 ml)	235
Yogurt (5 oz/150 g)	225
Broccolini (raw) (2½ oz/80 g)	160
Spinach, dandelion greens, or curly kale (steamed) (3½ oz /100 g)	150
Okra (raw) (2½ oz /80 g)	130
Cottage cheese, low-fat (3½ oz /100 g)	125
Soy yogurt (calcium-fortified) (110 g)	120
Shrimp (raw or boiled) (3½ oz /100 g)	110

Food	Calcium (mg)
Tofu (3½ oz/100 g)*	100*
Baked beans (½ can) (7½ oz /210 g)	100
Red kidney beans (½ drained can/ 4 oz /120 g)	85
Dried figs (1 oz /30 g)	80
Whole wheat bread (2 medium slices) (2½ oz /80 g)	75
Orange (5½ oz /160 g)	75
Almonds (1 oz /30 g)	70
Watercress (1 oz /30 g)	50
Broccoli (raw) (2½ oz /80 g)	45
Sweet potato (raw or cooked) (6 oz /180 g)	45
Cabbage (raw or cooked) (2½ oz /80 g)	40
Peas (fresh or frozen) (2½ oz /80 g)	30
Green beans and French beans (raw or cooked) (2½ oz /80 g)	30
Egg	30
Rhubarb (stewed), 3 tablespoons (2½ oz /80 g)	30
Apricots or currants (dried) (1 oz /30 g)	30
Red lentils (dried) (1½ oz /45 g)	25

* The amount of calcium in tofu varies widely among brands. Make sure you choose tofu that has been set with calcium and contains calcium in the ingredients.

How to eat less salt

Too much salt can have a damaging effect on your health—it can raise your blood pressure, putting you at higher risk of heart disease and stroke, and encourage loss of calcium from the bones, increasing the risk of osteoporosis. Current guidelines recommend no more than 2,300 mg per day (about a teaspoon)—yet the average person in the UK consumes 3,400 mg per day.[8] Many experts believe that we would be healthier if we cut down to just 1,500 mg per day. About three-quarters of salt is hidden in the food we buy, especially processed foods such as frozen meals, canned soups, sausages, pizzas, and takeout. When buying food, check the label for the salt content per 100 g—low salt is less than 120 mg salt or 0.1 g sodium.

How to cut down your salt intake

- Limit your intake of frozen meals and ready-made sauces.
- Cut down on salty snacks such as potato chips and salted nuts.
- Avoid adding extra salt while cooking or at the table. Flavor with black pepper, fresh or dried herbs, or lemon juice instead.
- Choose reduced-salt versions of baked beans and soups.
- Choose canned vegetables and beans in water.
- Limit your intake of salty fish, such as kippers and smoked salmon, and salty meat products such as bacon and ham.

A word on food labeling

It's always good to know what is in the food you buy, especially when you're following a diet. You don't need to count calories on The 2-Day Diet, but you may want to check food labels.

Nutrition Facts Label

DVs, or Daily Values, indicate the approximate amount of nutrients or calories that an average person requires for a healthy diet. The nutrition facts label (or nutrition information panel) can be found on the back of most packaged food. It lists the percentage supplied of important nutrients, usually based on a daily diet of 2,000 calories. The label begins with a standard serving measure, the servings per package, and calories per serving; always listed are total fat, sodium, carbohydrates, and protein. Usually all the following are listed: calories, calories from fat, fat, saturated fat, transfat, cholesterol, sodium, total carbohydrates, dietary fiber, sugar, protein, vitamin A, vitamin C, calcium, and iron. Not all beneficial nutrients are listed; for example, most labels will not include the amount of nutrients like omega-3 fats, or micronutrients.

Your questions answered

What about transfats?

Transfats are fats that naturally occur in small amounts in meat. Until recently, the main dietary source of transfats was manufactured foods containing unsaturated fats that had been processed (hydrogenated) to become saturated. This was done to help solidify and preserve foods such as margarines, cookies, cakes, potato chips, and crackers.

Transfats are bad for our health and have been linked to heart disease. Thankfully, as a result of pressure from consumers and the government, many manufacturers have removed transfats from foods in the US. They are still present in some products, though, so check the nutrition label and avoid foods that have

hydrogenated or partially hydrogenated vegetable oil or short-
ening listed in the ingredients.

Should I be sticking to low-GI foods?

Some diets focus on low-glycemic-index (GI) foods as a
way to lose weight, and you will see GI ratings on some food
labels. A food's GI score measures how quickly blood sugar
rises when you eat that food and applies only to carbohydrates.
Foods such as meat and cheese don't have a GI rating. The GI
of foods is ranked from 0 to 100 (with sugar at 100).

High-GI foods are broken down rapidly and raise the blood
sugar quickly, while low-GI foods are digested slowly and gradually release sugar into the bloodstream. However, to make
matters more complicated, the impact of the food on blood
sugar depends not just on its GI, but also the amount of
carbohydrate it contains (known as the glycemic load). Some
foods with a high GI, such as watermelon (GI 72), contain
very little carbohydrate so will have a minimal effect on blood
sugar. On top of that, the GI of carbohydrate foods tells you
only what happens when the food is eaten in isolation, and this
rarely happens—the GI is lowered, for example, when carbohydrate foods are eaten in combination with protein and fat. In
addition, not all low-GI foods are healthy—chocolate and ice
cream, for example, have a low GI! It can be extremely confus-
ing, so our recommendation is to forget GI—just aim to have
a high-fiber diet and unrefined foods.

Are sweeteners safe?

There are two main types of sweetener. Intense sweeteners
such as aspartame and sucralose are far sweeter than sugar
and tend to be used in soft drinks. There is some concern that
they may increase appetite and upset the beneficial balance

of intestinal bacteria, although this is still unclear. Bulk sweeteners such as xylitol and sorbitol contain half the calories of sugar and are used in sweet foods to add volume and texture as well as sweetness. High doses of these can cause symptoms of nausea and diarrhea and may also upset the balance of intestinal bacteria, although more research is needed. Any sweetener used in food in the US has to undergo safety testing and have an agreed acceptable daily intake level (ADI), which incorporates a safety margin.

Although the current guideline for aspartame is to consume less than 40 mg daily—equivalent to about 12 cans of a diet drink—the findings of two recent studies raise concerns that aspartame may be linked with certain blood cancers, which has sounded a note of caution with respect to their use. The links were seen both in animal studies, where consumption was equivalent to six cans of diet drinks per day, and in a population study in which intakes of up to three quarts of diet drinks per week were linked to higher rates of blood cancers in men but not in women.[9] Although these are preliminary findings, it makes sense to limit your intake of diet drinks to no more than three quarts—i.e., eight 12-oz cans of diet drinks per week (see page 56). Don't be tempted to replace diet drinks with sugary drinks, which are bad for both your health and your weight. In the above study, sugary drinks were as strongly linked to blood cancer as diet drinks.

Am I allowed any alcohol?

You can have an occasional alcoholic drink, but try not to drink more than seven units a week, and none on the two restricted days of The 2-Day Diet (see table on page 87 to see how many units of alcohol are in a typical drink). Alcohol

delivers double trouble for the dieter. It's packed with calories—an 8½ fl oz (250 ml) glass of wine contains 260 calories
and a standard "alcopop" 200 calories—and it makes you less
inhibited, so you are more likely to give in to the temptation
to eat! We know that alcohol consumed before or with meals
makes you eat more. Even an aperitif can increase intake by
30 percent.[10] While drinking a little may help protect against
heart disease, alcohol can increase the risk of several different
cancers, including breast, bowel, liver, mouth, and esopha-
geal cancer. The best choice, with fewest calories, is a spirit
plus a diet mixer (for example, gin and diet tonic, whiskey
and diet cola, or vodka and diet lemonade). Decide on the
maximum you are going to drink before you go out for the
evening. Start with a low-cal soft drink or water and avoid
salty snacks, which make you thirsty (and are usually full of
calories). Try to drink more low-cal soft drinks or sparkling
water than alcohol.

Alcohol	Units	Calories
Glass of wine 13% (8½ fl oz/250 ml)	3.3	240
Cider (1 pint/568 ml bottle)	2.3	210
Pint of beer/lager 4% (1 pint/568 ml)	2.3	170
Glass of wine 13% (6 fl oz/175 ml)	2.3	170
Champagne (4 fl oz/125 ml)	1.5	100
Alcopop 5% (9 fl oz/275 ml bottle)	1.4	200
Port (1¾ fl oz/50 ml)	1	79
Sherry (1¾ fl oz/50 ml)	1	58
Gin and diet tonic (1 fl oz/25 ml gin)	1	50

Should I cut out caffeine?

Many people assume that decaffeinated tea or coffee is "healthier" and that caffeine may raise blood pressure and increase the risk of heart disease. In fact, there's no evidence that tea and coffee, caffeinated or otherwise, are bad for your health. Both can be a satisfying drink that can fend off the urge for a snack. Experts agree that for most people there is no clear association between caffeine consumption and the risk of high blood pressure or heart disease,[11] although for people with high blood pressure, caffeine might cause a further slight temporary increase. Both tea and coffee are packed with disease-fighting antioxidants, which can lower your risk of heart disease and certain cancers. And as long as you are getting enough calcium, caffeine isn't bad for bones: in fact, the polyphenols in tea and coffee may actually be protective.

You might prefer to drink decaf, because caffeinated drinks stop some people from sleeping. Decaffeinated versions still contain beneficial antioxidants, and there are no obvious concerns with the chemicals used in the decaffeination process.

It does, however, make sense to limit your intake of tea, coffee, and other caffeinated drinks to no more than half your total drinks during the day, because they are diuretics, so they make you produce more urine and lose water. A recent review concluded that it is safe to consume 400 mg of caffeine per day with no adverse effects. Pregnant women should consume no more than 200 mg of caffeine per day (see following box), while children should consume no more than 1.25 mg per lb body weight/day.[12]

What is your caffeine intake?

- 1 mug of brewed coffee (125 mg)
- 1 mug of instant coffee (100 mg)
- 1 mug of tea (65 mg)
- 1 can of diet cola drink (40 mg)
- 1 oz (30 g) of 70% plain chocolate (24 mg)

Is it safe to eat oily fish?

Fish is good for you and is an important part of your 2-Day Diet—especially oily fish, which is one of our few dietary sources of vitamin D. However, current advice from the FDA and EPA is to avoid or limit certain types of fish because they contain mercury, which can be harmful. These include swordfish, tilefish, shark, king mackerel, and orange roughy. Children and women who are pregnant or planning to become pregnant should also avoid these fish completely. You can safely eat unlimited amounts of fish such as cod, snapper, skate, pollock, squid, Dover sole, dab, flounder, tilapia, salmon, and white crabmeat.

Can I still have treats?

We found that our 2-Day Dieters fell into two groups—those who were eager to include treats as part of the Diet because they made it feel less restrictive and those who felt that it was important to cut out chocolate and other sweet snacks. Only you will know what works for you, but remember that restricting a food can lead to cravings and wanting to binge on it. If you want to include some treats as part of your Diet, we recommend limiting them to three servings a week (see the table on page 90). Note that some foods that are often thought

of as healthy, such as granola bars, are very high in calories—
so a "treat" is only two minibites (1-in/3-cm square).

If you don't think you can live without chocolate, don't
worry. Although you can't have chocolate on your two
restricted days of The 2-Day Diet, it's fine to have a bit of
chocolate, or another "treat" food during the five unrestricted
days. Chocolate is high in calories, sugar, and saturated fat, so
don't overdo it (see below for recommended amounts) and
choose a dark chocolate that's high in cocoa solids (70–85
percent) that may help reduce blood pressure and improve
blood sugar control. In fact, a recent study allocated women
to eat either 20 g (⅔ oz) of 80 percent dark chocolate a day
or 20 g (⅔ oz) of standard milk chocolate every day for four
weeks. The good news was that women eating the 80 percent
chocolate saw a reduction in their blood pressure and insulin
levels; however, the milk chocolate group saw quite the oppo-
site effect, and these women had a 20 percent reduction in
the efficiency of their insulin.[13]

Treat	Servings
Low-fat potato chips	1 small packet (¾–1 oz/25–30 g)
Plain or chocolate graham crackers or small oatmeal cookies	2
Chocolate (ideally dark > 70% cocoa)	5 small squares or 1 oz (30 g)
Ice cream	2 scoops (3½ oz/100 g) standard or 1 scoop (1¾ oz/50 g) luxury
Fruit bread	1 slice
Mini cupcakes	2 small cakes with thin or no icing
Granola bar	½ bar
Small chocolate chip cookies	3
Individual chocolate or truffle	3

Snack ideas for the five unrestricted days of the week

- Whole grain crackers or rye crisps with low-fat hummus, low-fat cream cheese, or low-fat cottage cheese.
- Fruit.
- Vegetable crudités, such as celery, cucumber, green peppers, snow peas, scallions, and cherry tomatoes with salsa, low-fat hummus, tzatziki, or guacamole.
- Plain, diet, or fruit yogurt.
- Small handful of unsalted nuts (i.e., walnuts, pistachios, or Brazil nuts) or dried fruit (e.g., apricots, figs, golden raisins, or mangoes).
- A glass of vegetable juice (carrot, tomato, or mixture).
- Plain popcorn (popped in vegetable oil with no sugar or salt added).
- Bowl of soup (see pages 249–255).
- Smoothie made with fat-free or 1% milk, yogurt, and one piece of fruit.
- Dried pea snacks.
- Sugar-free jelly.
- Popsicle made from frozen, diluted sugar-free fruit-flavored drink.

Summary

▶ The five unrestricted days of The 2-Day Diet are based on a healthy Mediterranean diet with lots of vegetables, whole grains, beans, fish, fruit, nuts, and healthy oils and can include small amounts of lean red meat.

▶ Eating foods that are high in soluble and insoluble fiber will help keep you full and keep your blood sugar stable and your bowels healthy.

▶ Make sure you still have plenty of healthy protein foods on the five unrestricted days of The 2-Day Diet, as this will help to fill you up and stop you from overeating. This will maximize your weight loss with The 2-Day Diet.

▶ Low-fat dairy foods help fill you up and keep your bones strong.

▶ It's important to stay well hydrated and to drink at least eight glasses of fluid a day.

▶ You are allowed occasional treats, such as alcohol and chocolate, but limit them to two or three times a week.

5

making The 2-Day Diet work

You've made the decision to start The 2-Day Diet and you're on your way. The focus of this chapter is to lay the groundwork that will make sure you have the best chance of success, help you to deal with any problems that might arise, and answer your diet questions.

Eight steps to successful weight loss

Step one: plan ahead

Prepare a shopping list before you set out to do your weekly shopping—and stick to it. If you have the right foods at home, you're more likely to persevere with The 2-Day Diet, but if your cabinets are stuffed with temptations like cookies, potato chips, and chocolate, you will be making your life much harder. "Out of sight" really is "out of mind," and craving-inducing comfort foods are much easier to avoid if they aren't around to tempt you. One study found that simply moving dishes of candies from people's desks to the other side of the room meant that they ate less of them.[1] If you keep snacks in the cabinet "for the kids" and often end up digging into them yourself, ask yourself whether it's time to get these snacks out of the house and improve the children's diets too. If not (if you can't face the mutiny!), store them in a special container marked "Kids only!"

Try the following tips:

▶ Never go food shopping on an empty stomach: it is too tempting to buy (and then eat) things that you'll regret later.

▶ Pack a healthy homemade lunch to take to work and keep healthy snacks (if you're likely to need them) in your office drawer, handbag, or car to help you avoid the temptation of eating things that you shouldn't. For ideas, see the meal plans in chapter 8 (pages 169–178).

▶ Don't be afraid to let people know that you're trying to lose weight and would prefer not to have chocolate, candy, or cakes as gifts, or for them to persuade you to indulge if you meet them for a coffee.

▶ Ask your friends and family to actively support your weight-loss efforts (see page 36). Talk it up and let the important people in your life know how you're doing and feeling. If you're struggling and need some encouragement, don't beat around the bush—just ask for it.

▶ Find us on Facebook to connect with other 2-Day Dieters and to share your experiences.

I've always had a thing for pastry, chocolate, and cakes,
and the lack of them is the only negative about the diet.
But I'm adapting well now that I understand the effects
they are having on my body and my health. —Susie, 35

Step two: watch your liquid calories

Drinks can work for or against you. Having a glass of water
or another noncalorie drink when you are eating a meal has
been shown to reduce the amount you eat,[2] but some drinks
are loaded with calories. A 12 fl oz (330 ml) can of regular cola
contains 145 calories—whereas the diet version contains only
one calorie. What's more, these fluid calories bypass normal
appetite controls, making it all too easy to consume too many.
If you need carbonated drinks in your life, include an occasional diet soda in your eating plan. Despite some concerns,
there's no convincing evidence that these can increase osteoporosis risk by leaching calcium from the bones as long as you
are getting enough calcium in your diet.

The same applies to other drinks—a couple of lattes can
really bump up your calorie count, even if you go for the skinny
version. A large full-fat milk latte comes in at a whopping 223
calories, while the fat-free milk version still contains 131 calories. By contrast, an Americano with 1% milk contains only 20
calories, so drink coffee or tea with a splash of milk or herbal
teas instead.

Step three: beware of portion distortion

Most of us have noticed that serving sizes have grown massively
over the last few decades and are getting larger as food companies and outlets want to sell us more food, and we have become
used to these larger portions. Twenty years ago a medium slice
of bread weighed 1 oz (30 g) and contained 65 calories; today

it weighs 1½ oz (45 g) and contains 90 calories. Similarly, coffee shop muffins have grown in size from 1½ oz to 4 oz and from 210 to 500 calories.

Many high-calorie snack foods are two, or even three, times as big as they were 30 years ago—and that means twice or three times the calories. Researchers have shown that when we are presented with servings that are bigger than we need, most of us will eat more without even thinking about it.[3] The good news is that, conversely, if we're given smaller servings and fewer calories, we will eat less without feeling deprived.[4] That's why, as well as telling you the types of food to eat, The 2-Day Diet provides clear guidelines on the amounts to eat for dieting success. This should not be an issue on the two restricted days of The 2-Day Diet, when the high-protein foods mean that you tend to self-limit what you eat. We certainly don't expect you to weigh all your foods—we provide simple guidelines for gauging portion sizes alongside weights of food servings both on the two restricted days and on the five unrestricted days of The 2-Day Diet. Many of our 2-Day Dieters did find it helpful to weigh foods such as breakfast cereals, pasta, and rice, which are easy to pour out and overdo, until they got used to the recommended serving sizes.

Being able to vary the restricted days of The 2-Day Diet means I can fit them around social occasions and holidays, so I don't feel as though I'm missing out. —Jane, 49

Step four: sit at a table to eat

Eating on the run, or while you are watching TV, sitting at your desk, at your computer, or even listening to the radio, means that you are focusing on something else, and you will tend to consume more calories—simply because you don't notice what or how much you are eating.[5] In one study, people eating potato chips while watching TV ate around 40 percent more than on another occasion when they didn't watch any TV.[6]

The best way to avoid uncontrolled munching is to sit down at a table, eat slowly, and savor each mouthful—without doing something else, such as watching TV, at the same time. It takes about 15 minutes for your brain to let your stomach know that you have eaten enough, so make yourself wait at least 15 minutes after finishing a meal to decide whether you are still hungry and whether you really need seconds or dessert.

> *The 2-Day Diet suited me, as it taught me to eat the correct food types and experiment with different foods. I've been losing the inches. Trousers that were tight are now comfortable, and I don't get that bloated feeling.*
> —Ruth, 53

Step five: avoid "diet" foods

The supermarkets are full of them—the low-fat, low-sugar "diet" foods that promise an easy way to eat fewer calories and lose weight. We don't recommend basing your diet on these highly processed diet foods, but to stick to the whole and unprocessed foods we recommend on the restricted and unrestricted days of The 2-Day Diet. Of course it can be helpful knowing the calorie content of foods. Don't forget that calories will be listed per serving, so you will need to multiply this to work out how many calories are in each package.

Don't mistake "low-fat" for "low-calorie." A lot of foods labeled "light," "lite," or "lower-fat" can still contain quite large amounts of fat and, therefore, calories. Manufacturers often replace the fat in low-fat foods with sugar to improve the flavor, so these foods can provide just as many calories and often contain fructose (see page 73). The only "diet" foods that may be useful are low-fat foods and those that use artificial sweeteners with no added sugar, such as diet drinks. Remember to stay within the limit of no more than three quarts (eight 12-oz cans) of diet drinks per week.

Step six: manage your expectations

Stick to the rules of The 2-Day Diet and follow the exercise guidelines (see chapter 6), and we promise you will achieve successful—and rapid—weight loss. That said, it won't happen overnight, and you might experience a few setbacks. You will be burning fat on the two restricted days of The 2-Day Diet, but you will notice a drop in your weight during and immediately afterward as you also lose water—typically between 1 and 2 lb (0.5 and 1 kg) over the two days. Fat burning is a complex process, and most people won't lose any more than 4½ lb (2 kg) of fat per week. Any weight loss beyond this will just be loss of water.

If you think back to how long it has taken you to put on your excess weight, you have to be realistic and realize that it will take a while to get rid of it too. A pound (0.5 kg) of body fat contains around 4,500 calories, so, in theory, to lose a pound of fat in a week, you should burn off or consume 4,500 fewer calories—around 640 fewer calories per day. Unfortunately, it's not that simple, because when you diet, your metabolic rate falls, and your body adapts to a lower calorie intake. Research that monitored calorie intake and expenditure (from resting metabolic rate and activity) and fat loss found that to lose one pound of fat per week, on average, you actually need to eat 850 calories less than you need each day.[7] This is a lot of calories to cut down on, and by far the best way to do it is through a combination of diet and exercise. If you do 30 minutes of exercise five times a week, you only need to eat 700 fewer calories per day to lose the weight. If you exercise for an hour five times a week, you would only have to eat 550 fewer calories. You might feel a bit disappointed by the fact that exercise burns so few calories, but remember that exercise improves overall health and reduces the risks of many diseases (see page 118). What's more, we consistently find that exercise appears to help Dieters adhere better to their weight-loss diet.

> *I am 30 years old and have lost just over 7 lb (3 kg) in three weeks. I noticed results within about a week. Every winter I always tend to grow my "winter coat" (i.e., put on a few pounds from eating comfort food!). This diet has really helped me to drop the weight, which I have been unable to lose through exercise and other diets.*
> —Sally, 30

Step seven: monitor your progress

Monitoring is a vital part of any weight-loss plan. We know that dieters who monitor themselves do better. The way you feel in your clothes will give you clues about what's happening to your weight, but you should still weigh yourself, measure your waist and hips once a week, and make a note of the results. You can use these measurements to reassess your percentage of body fat and weight of body fat—ideally every two weeks—using the calculator in Appendix A (pages 313–314).

How to monitor yourself

- Weight can fluctuate from day to day (up or down by 2–4½ lb/1–2 kg), so it is not a good idea to weigh yourself every day, as this could give you a skewed picture of your overall progress.

- Weight can change throughout the day, so always weigh and measure yourself at the same time of day (ideally first thing in the morning, as we are usually heavier at the end of the day) and before eating a meal.

- Use the same set of reliable scales. Don't stand bathroom scales on an uneven or soft surface such as a carpet—most bathroom scales work best when placed on a hard, level floor.

- Remove your clothes and shoes before weighing yourself, or wear light layers only.

- Measure your waist and hips without clothes on, as some clothes can be constricting and give unreliable, sometimes misleading, measurements.

- For women, weight and waist measurements are often greater just before your period because of fluid retention—you may see gains of 4½ lb (2 kg), even up to 11 lb (5 kg), depending on how much you weigh.

- Because you will lose water on the two restricted days of The 2-Day Diet, we suggest that you weigh yourself immediately before and not after your restricted days each week. If you step on the scales immediately after the two days, you will be lighter, as you will have lost fluid as well as some fat.

*I eat out a lot, and in the past restaurants have always
been the scene of my diet-breaking crimes, but it's
definitely been possible to choose from a normal menu—
even on a restricted day. I've probably had to eat out on
at least one of my two restricted days each week since I
started the diet, and I'm still seeing brilliant results. This
has to be the easiest diet to fit around your real life.*
—Alison, 26

Step eight: reward your success

Although your final reward—reaching your weight-loss goal—
is some way down the line, it's important to recognize and
reward yourself for even small successes on the way. Losing
weight takes focus and commitment, and you deserve regular
pats on the back for your hard work. You should have already
set yourself short-term weight-loss and exercise goals. Setting
up a reward system adds an extra incentive, prevents you from
getting bored, and gives you something to work toward.

Rewards are a very personal thing, and only you know
what would be a real treat for you—although treats should
obviously not involve food or alcohol! This could be your
opportunity to use the money you've saved on The 2-Day
Diet to treat yourself (see page 68). Buy yourself some new
clothes or that new pair of boots or shoes you've been long-
ing for; arrange to have a facial, manicure, pedicure, or new
haircut; book a day off work and just take it easy; reserve tick-
ets for a film, play, or show that you want to see. For men, why
not go for a spin on the go-kart track or get that new gizmo
for your toolbox that you've been hankering after?

CASE STUDY: Sarah

At over 200 lb (91 kg) Sarah was desperate to lose weight. Her mother had been diagnosed with breast cancer in her forties, and 10 years later the cancer had come back. A self- confessed chocoholic, Sarah, 39, knew that being overweight increased her risk of breast cancer. She tried weight-loss clubs and many different diets at home, but although she lost some weight, it always piled back on. By the time Sarah started The 2-Day Diet she had almost given up hope. "I knew it would be a challenge, but I developed a routine, making the same two days each week my diet days and eating the same foods each week. I made the diet days my busiest workdays so that I didn't miss eating. What surprised me was that I didn't want to overeat on my nondiet days—perhaps because I had become more aware of what I was eating. I lost 14 lb (6.4 kg) in the first month and over a six-month period lost 56 lb (25.5 kg). It is the easiest diet I have ever done."

Your questions answered

Is it important to eat at particular times of the day?

When we eat is dictated by all sorts of things—family habits, social pressure, and convenience—as well as actually feeling hungry. There is no conclusive evidence that eating earlier in the day, avoiding eating after a certain time in the evening, or having smaller, more frequent meals rather than large meals will have any impact on your metabolic rate and your body's ability to burn or store fat.[8] However, what *is* important is your individual response to the timing and the frequency of eating that may make you prone to overeating in certain situations. If you know that evenings are a time when you get the munchies, or that you find it hard not to eat a large dinner even if you aren't hungry, then it's important to become aware of this and to take precautions for times when you might overeat. Evenings are danger times for many people, and it often helps to stay busy—for example, you could sort out the newspapers, do the ironing, or do something practical with your hands (such as knitting) while watching TV. If tea and cookies in front of the TV is your "reward" after a hard day's work, but you can't stop at just one cookie, find another way to reward yourself—with a long aromatic bath or an evening out. It also helps to brush your teeth after the last time you eat during the day—to signal to your body that eating is over for the day.

Isn't eating after 5 p.m. more fattening?

Lots of people believe this, but science shows quite clearly that it's the total number of calories you consume over the 24 hours that determines whether you gain or lose weight. Food eaten in the evening is *no* more likely to be stored as fat than food eaten earlier in the day. A number of studies have found that food eaten late at night is processed in exactly the same way as the same food eaten as several small meals throughout the day.[9]

I've heard that lack of sleep can make you fat. Does it?

We all have an internal body clock, which is controlled by our brain and which helps coordinate the hormones that control our appetite and the metabolism of food. Our body clocks are designed to function around our normal pattern of waking and sleeping, which, in turn, is fundamentally controlled by the cycle of daylight and darkness. If our lifestyle is at odds with this body clock, it can affect our metabolism and weight control. Although this is a new area of research, there is emerging evidence that if you are someone who has less sleep and prefers to be up at night and eat most of your food at night, or someone who has to do this because of shift work, you could be at a greater risk of gaining weight due to increased appetite and possibly reductions in your metabolic rate and fat burning.

Research consistently shows that having only five to six hours' sleep increases the appetite and daily calorie intake by 200 calories.[10] In a recent study conducted in a hotel-type setting in Boston, volunteers spent three weeks in conditions where they were allowed only five and a half hours' sleep per night. Their body clocks were disrupted through being denied daylight and being put onto a 28-hour cycle. After just three weeks, their resting metabolic rate fell by 8 percent—a drop that would translate into weight gain of around 13 lb (5.8 kg) over a year.[11]

If you are a shift worker

Working shifts and dieting to lose weight takes more planning and self-discipline than if you work normal hours because some disruption to your body clock is inevitable. But it can be done—the recent brilliantly titled Australian POWER (Preventing Obesity Without Eating like a Rabbit!) study asked a group of male shift workers in an aluminum plant to follow a healthy calorie-controlled diet and included exercise using the tips on page 105. It worked! After 14 weeks the men had lost, on average, nearly 9 lb (4 kg) and 1½ in (4 cm) from their waists.[12]

Tips for shift workers

- If you work nights, eat a light meal during the night and a small breakfast when you finish work.
- Plan ahead to help yourself eat as healthily as possible, especially in situations where the food available tends to be high-calorie greasy junk food. Take fruit and vegetables with you to snack on during your shift, and limit your intake of carbonated and caffeinated drinks. Drink water throughout your shift.
- Shift workers often struggle to get good-quality sleep. Make sure your bedroom is quiet, dark, and not too warm. Close the curtains or blinds, and wear earplugs and an eye mask if necessary. Make sure your family and friends know that this is your "night" and that you shouldn't be interrupted. Create a sleep schedule for yourself and stick to it, sleeping at the same time during the working week and on the weekends.
- Incorporate exercise into your breaks at work. Walk for 10 minutes and do some simple stretches.
- Fit cardiovascular and resistance exercises (see pages 122–123) into the time after you rest or wake up.
- Join a 24-hour gym if you want to work out during irregular hours. Run, walk, cycle, dance, or do any activity that gets your heart rate up and burns calories.
- Talk to other shift workers and share tips on how to stay healthy while working shifts. Create or join a support group with your peers.

Do I have to eat breakfast?

We've all been told that a good breakfast is essential for physical and mental performance, because your body hasn't been fed all night and it needs food to refuel. And it's often quoted as a vital meal for dieters, as it will kick-start your metabolism and help to control overeating later in the day. While it's important that children have their breakfast, our advice is, don't force yourself to eat breakfast if you don't want it. Some of us are "morning" people who feel hungry and need breakfast to get going, but if you can't face breakfast first thing and so tend not to eat it, follow your appetite and wait until you are hungry. When researchers from London's University of Roehampton asked men who didn't normally eat breakfast to include it, they didn't eat less for the rest of the day—in fact, they ate 300 calories more than normal. But when people who always ate breakfast were asked to skip it, they overate later in the day.[13] The take-home message is that we are probably all wired differently, so do what feels right for you. If you are a breakfast eater, it doesn't have to be toast and cereal—a high-protein breakfast, such as eggs, will help you feel fuller for longer. When researchers compared an egg-based, 400-calorie breakfast with a 400-calorie carbohydrate-based breakfast (bagels in this case), the egg eaters consumed 400 fewer calories during the day than the bagel eaters.[14]

I have tried to lose weight so many times before that I don't know whether it's worth trying again. Has dieting messed up my metabolism?

We have found The 2-Day Diet to be successful, not just for first-time dieters, but for people who have tried time after time to lose weight. Some of our Dieters had more than 10 previous attempts at dieting. Researchers at the Fred Hutchinson Cancer Research Center in Seattle found that "yo-yo" dieters who had tried and failed to lose weight three or more times previously were just as able to lose weight and see

reductions in insulin and inflammation in the body (the antic-
ipated beneficial effect of weight loss) as dieters who hadn't
ever been on a diet.[15]

A word about snacking

To snack or not to snack? It's a topic of endless debate. Some
people argue that snacking helps to control your appetite
because it stops you getting really hungry and then overeating at
mealtimes. Others say that snacking just encourages you to keep
focusing on food and makes you eat more. We often see dieters
who have previously tried to eat something religiously every hour
or so, believing it will boost their metabolism, although this is not
the case.

    There is no evidence that snacking between meals is better
for controlling hunger or reducing levels of "appetite" hormones.
And there is no difference in your metabolic rate whether you
eat two large meals or six or seven smaller ones a day if you
consume the same amount overall. It's possible that you may
burn less body fat after a large meal, but the impact of this will
be extremely small.[16]

    At the end of the day, how many meals you eat really depends
on you, and the bottom line is not when you eat, but how much
you eat in total within the 24-hour day. You probably know the
pattern of eating that suits you best and helps control your appetite. If not, experiment with it and see whether it works better for
you to stick with two or three large meals or to have five or six
smaller ones.

    It might be worth remembering that as long as you don't over-
eat, there may actually be health benefits in leaving longer periods
between eating. We know that beneficial changes occur when our

cells are not constantly fed with calories (see page 18). So leaving longer gaps between meals, when your cells aren't being "fed," may have a beneficial effect. For most of us, this happens every night as we have 12 hours without food between our last meal of the day and breakfast—although it may not happen if you are up snacking in front of the TV until 2 a.m. and eat a big breakfast at 7 a.m. when you get up.

SWAP IT! See how many calories you could save!

✘	✔
Can of cola and chocolate muffin (465 calories)	Diet cola and apple (45 calories)
Bar of milk chocolate (280 calories)	Diet yogurt (100 calories)
Bag of potato chips (160 calories)	Vegetable sticks and low-calorie dip (25 calories)

Help—I've broken my diet!

Even the most dedicated dieter slips up from time to time—and the slipup is usually eating "forbidden" foods. This is one reason why we have made sure there are treats on The 2-Day Diet! If you do slip up, don't beat yourself up about it or feel like a failure—and certainly don't give up. Dieting lapses happen to everyone, and the best thing you can do is to get back on track as soon as you can. For our 2-Day Dieters, holidays were the biggest danger times. Some also struggled when they were stressed, short of time, premenstrual, or when they found themselves in certain social situations. Even though you are unrestricted for five days out of seven each week, there may be times when it is helpful to prescribe yourself a diet "break," which can be a good way to deal with high-risk periods or to combat diet boredom. One recent study looked at the impact of a planned two-week diet "break" on people's long-term success. The result? After the break, the dieters managed to successfully return to their diets and it did not hamper their long-term success.[17] If you know that you have an event or a special occasion coming up, think ahead and plan to deviate from the Diet temporarily and then get back on track afterward—rather than convincing yourself that you will not be tempted on the day and then being disappointed with yourself when you do.

Don't forget, if you do lapse, try to learn from the experience to enable yourself to avoid doing the same thing the next time. Ask yourself: "What was the situation?" "How did I respond?" "How did I feel afterward?" and "What could I do differently next time?"

Why is my weight loss slowing down?

Weight loss becomes harder when you have been dieting for a while, usually after about six months have gone by. Part of this may be due to the inevitable 10–15 percent reduction in metabolic rate that happens as your body adapts to weight loss and eating less (even when you exercise). But weight loss often slows down because you may not be sticking as carefully to the Diet or exercising as much as when you first started.

If you feel you are not losing the predicted 1–2 lb (0.5–1 kg) per week, check the following:

▶ Are you following the correct diet plan for someone of your sex, weight, and age (see Appendix D, pages 327–335)?

▶ Are you overeating on the two restricted days of The 2-Day Diet?

▶ Are you overeating on the five unrestricted days of The 2-Day Diet or drinking too much alcohol?

▶ Are you doing the recommended amount of exercise (see chapter 6)?

▶ Are you taking every opportunity to be physically active in your daily routine—for example, taking the stairs or choosing to walk rather than drive, where possible?

▶ Keep a tally of your food servings and record your activities for four days to check how much you are eating and how active you really are. Remember to include weekdays *and* weekends.

How do I beat my food cravings?

Most of us have foods that we crave occasionally. Unfortunately, when you are trying to diet, these cravings can become worse. Although some cravings are driven by hunger, many are triggered by internal cues—if you feel bored or anxious, you might be in the habit of eating chocolate to make yourself feel better. You may also respond to external cues, such as chocolate by the cash register when you are buying your healthy salad lunch, other people eating, or certain social situations. Interestingly, many of our 2-Day Dieters stopped craving chocolate and sweet treats but sometimes craved bread, cereals, and other carbohydrates on their two restricted days, which of course they were then able to eat on their five unrestricted days.

Try to identify your particular triggers. When are you most likely to feel those cravings, and what are the common factors? Is it about the way you feel, what is happening around you, or a combination of the two? The good news is that you can reprogram your brain to overcome these urges. You may just have a craving to eat something—in which case try having a hot drink, a diet drink, or perhaps some sugar-free mints or sugar-free chewing gum.

There are two approaches that can be helpful:

▶ **Distraction.** A food craving is like a wave that gets bigger and bigger but then subsides. So while a craving can feel overwhelming—and irresistible—as it builds up, you need to remind yourself that it will pass. Try to ride it out by distracting yourself. You may find that the craving will go if you can distract yourself for 15 to 20 minutes by focusing on something else. Get busy with housework, phone a friend, go for a walk, have a shower, or clean your teeth.

▶ **Acceptance** (feel the craving and work through it). Let yourself experience the full force of the craving, be really conscious of it, and try to notice what you are thinking and feeling without giving in to it. This approach may be harder initially, but learning that you can manage to resist the urge to eat the food you crave can give you a real sense of achievement and make it easier next time, because you know that you are able to take control and make choices about what you eat.[18]

How can I stop myself from comfort-eating?

Many of us overeat when we are stressed or depressed. Although eating can give you a quick fix, in the longer term comfort eating doesn't provide much comfort, especially if you're trying to lose weight, and it often leaves you feeling more anxious and stressed. The key here is to recognize when you are stressed and find ways to manage it (see page 38).

I always get the munchies before my period. What should I do?

The week before the start of a period is a difficult time for many women. As well as feeling moody and anxious, women commonly experience cravings, especially for high-carbohydrate foods. It's thought that these cravings are due to your body trying to take in enough carbohydrate to balance levels of chemicals in the brain.

About half our Dieters had difficulty managing premenstrual syndrome (PMS) cravings on the two restricted days of The 2-Day Diet. We suggest that you experiment and see how you feel. If it's too difficult to do your two restricted days when you are premenstrual, try to reschedule these days for when you're not suffering from PMS.

Try to deal with carbohydrate cravings on the five unrestricted eating days by eating whole grain rather than refined carbohydrates (see page 74). Calcium, magnesium, and vitamin B_6 are all thought to help reduce PMS and suppress cravings,[19] so eat plenty of foods rich in these nutrients. Calcium is found in low-fat dairy foods, eggs, spinach, green vegetables, canned sardines, and salmon (including the bones). Some good dietary sources of magnesium include whole grain cereals and vegetables. Good sources of B_6 include lean meat, eggs, whole grain cereals, soybeans, peanuts, and milk.

The good news is that many women find that their PMS improves when they lose weight and do regular exercise.

I am prone to suffering from seasonal affective disorder (SAD) in winter. How can I curb my cravings?

Many of us get a touch of the "winter blues," when we feel low and lethargic during the winter months, but as much as 5 percent of people in the US suffer more severely and have what is known as seasonal affective disorder (SAD). This is caused by the lack of daylight affecting the chemical balance of the brain and reducing levels of serotonin, a chemical that promotes relaxation and happiness. SAD is more common among women, particularly those between ages 20 and 50. Whether you have the winter blues or full-blown SAD, you will probably notice a craving for starchy and sugary foods, which both help boost levels of serotonin in the brain. So what is the answer? Exercise is a great therapy, as it helps to restore the chemical balance of the brain and helps you to feel good about yourself. Walking outside for an hour a day has also been shown to help SAD sufferers.

We often find that people do better at losing weight in the summer, perhaps because low-calorie foods are more desirable and it's less tempting to have stodgy "comfort" foods when the weather is warm and it's easier to get out and exercise. In the summer, our Dieters lost, on average, 15 lb (6.8 kg), whereas in the winter, it was only 11½ lb (5.3 kg). This doesn't mean that you should delay starting your diet (and exercise) until the summer. Just be aware that losing weight in winter may be more of a challenge—and if you do delay, this may mean another winter when you gain weight, so you eventually have more to lose when you do start dieting.

Eating out and takeout

There will inevitably be times during your 2-Day Diet when you have to eat away from home because of work or social occasions. So how do you keep your 2-Day Diet on track?

- Meals out are usually bigger and higher in calories than meals at home, and they often contain lots of hidden fat. However, more restaurants and takeout outlets are now informing customers about the calorie content of their foods, to help make people more aware of the healthier choices. So do make use of this information if it is available. Try to avoid fixed-price menus as you may well end up eating more courses and calories than you need or want—just because it's included in the price. Also, "all you can eat" restaurants are probably best avoided—the temptation to pile your plate high just because you can is possibly too great!
- Don't starve yourself all day before you go out—you could overeat when you eventually sit down to your meal.
- Share courses with your companions so you don't overeat.
- Perhaps order just two starters instead of a starter plus a main course.
- Eat slowly and savor every mouthful.
- Don't be afraid to ask for exactly what you want by requesting that the menu is adapted. Most restaurants will be happy to do this.
- Ask for high-calorie sauces or dressings to be served on the side so that you can decide how much of them to put on your food.
- Don't be afraid to ask how the food is cooked if it is not clear from reading the menu. Most waiters are only too happy to explain these details.
- Be careful about eating lots of nibbles before the meal, such as bread soaked in olive oil or tortilla chips and guacamole, as they add lots of extra calories.

- Drink plenty of water and less wine. Ordinary tap water should be freely available and will save money on your drinks bill, as well as keeping your calories down.

- The following words and phrases mean that extra fat and calories have been added: à la crème, au gratin, battered, béarnaise, béchamel, beurre blanc, breaded, butter, crispy, cheese sauce, cordon bleu, creamed, en croûte, flaky, florentine, fried, hollandaise, meunière, Milanese, pan-fried, Parmesan, rich, sauté, scalloped, tempura.

Summary

▶ Plan ahead, monitor your weight loss and exercise, and control your serving sizes to give yourself the best chance of success.

▶ Find the pattern of eating that works for you, whether it's eating a few large meals or several smaller ones each day.

▶ Successful weight loss takes time. Don't be disheartened if the weight doesn't fall off as quickly as you had hoped or if it slows down. If you keep to The 2-Day Diet, you will succeed.

▶ Make sure you get enough sleep and manage your stress levels, as neglecting either can put you off track.

▶ Reward yourself for every success and don't be disappointed if things occasionally go wrong—just get back on The 2-Day Diet.

Cutting back on my bread and potatoes means that I don't feel so stodged up. My stomach has shrunk, so I don't feel so hungry. —Georgina, 53

6

how to be more active

Getting moving and staying active will speed up your weight loss, enhance the health benefits of The 2-Day Diet, and boost your mood and energy levels. The good news is that if you've been a confirmed couch potato up until now, it's never too late to start moving, and being active really doesn't have to be hard. Our 2-Day Dieters showed us that even if you've never exercised before, you can make physical activity a regular part of your life. We will show you how to start slowly, build up gradually, and stay motivated so that you hit your weight-loss and fitness goals.

Why you need to get moving

Left to their own devices, people tend to move less, rather than more, when they start dieting. Research shows that activity levels can drop by around 40 percent when people go on a diet, and when you move less you need fewer calories, which makes it harder to lose weight.[1] Get moving and it will have the reverse effect, increasing your weight loss, boosting your health, and helping you to look and feel better.

You'll lose more weight

When you lose weight, your metabolic rate falls because your body needs fewer calories in order to function. Exercise helps to combat this and keep your weight loss on track by burning extra calories. Exercise alone won't shift much extra weight— it's the combination of diet and exercise that really makes the difference. Research studies have shown that people who only exercise and don't diet lose only 3 lb (1.4 kg) and that those who only diet and don't exercise lose 16½ lb (7.5 kg); the real winners are those who diet and exercise— they shed 21 lb (9.5 kg).[2]

You'll maintain calorie-burning muscle

Everyone loses muscle as well as fat when they lose weight, but exercise can halve that muscle loss. So if you lose 19 lb (8.6 kg), you will lose 6 lb (2.7 kg) of that as muscle if you're not exercising. With exercise, you'll only lose 3 lb (1.4 kg) of muscle. Hanging on to that extra muscle is important for fat burning because muscle burns seven times more calories than fat. One of the major effects of aging is loss of muscle: the average Western woman loses about ½ lb (0.3 kg) of muscle every year. Exercising while you diet will reduce the rate of the aging process and save you six years of normal muscle loss.

I was a bit worried that exercising on my restricted days would make me hungrier and make me struggle to keep to the diet. Actually, going swimming after work gives me a routine, keeps me on track, and avoids the evening munchies. —Pat, 54

Your body will love it!

Our bodies are designed to move—and when they don't, they suffer. Bones and muscles become weaker, and your heart and lungs become less efficient at pumping blood around your body. Becoming active can actually boost your immune system, helping to protect you against viral infections and colds. A single exercise session can lower your blood pressure, increase the effectiveness of your insulin (this is called "insulin sensitivity"), and lower the levels of harmful fats in your blood for 24 to 48 hours.[3] Being active for 150 minutes a week—that's just half an hour five days a week—reduces your risk of type 2 diabetes, cuts heart disease and stroke risk by 30 percent, and cuts your risk of dying prematurely from any cause by 50 percent.[4] The health benefits of taking up exercise are considered as important as giving up smoking. Moving a bit more—three to four hours a week—can cut your risk of breast and colon cancer by 30 percent. On top of that, exercise will benefit your bones and joints, helping to protect you against osteoporosis and arthritis.

I always find I can keep to my diet better when I am also being active. A brisk walk or run can really boost my mood and make me determined not to overeat.
—Rachel, 44

Your mood will improve

You won't just feel the physical benefits of exercise—it can help to energize you, help you sleep better, alleviate depression, and stimulate the release of feel-good brain chemicals that help you feel happier and more relaxed. In fact, exercise combats many of the things that can make us overeat in the first place—stress, depression, and low self-esteem.

Getting started

However long it's been or however unfit you are, you *can* take the first step and commit yourself to becoming more active. The body never forgets how to adapt positively to exercise, even after several years of inactivity. Start by completing the physical activity readiness questionnaire (PAR-Q) below.

PAR-Q and You (A Questionnaire for People Aged 15 to 69)[5]

Regular physical activity is fun and healthy, and increasingly more people are starting to become more active every day. Being more active is very safe for most people. However, some people should check with their doctor before they start becoming much more physically active.

If you are planning to become much more physically active than you are now, start by answering the seven questions in the box below. If you are between the ages of 15 and 69, the PAR-Q will tell you if you should check with your doctor before you start. If you are over 69 years of age, and you are not used to being very active, check with your doctor.

Common sense is your best guide when you answer these questions. Please read the questions carefully and answer each one honestly: check YES or NO.

Has your doctor ever said that you have a heart condition and that you should only do physical activity recommended by them?

Yes ☐ No ☐

Do you feel pain in your chest when you do physical activity?

Yes ☐ No ☐

In the past month have you had chest pain when you were not doing physical activity?   Yes ☐ No ☐

Do you lose your balance because of dizziness or do you ever lose consciousness?   Yes ☐ No ☐

Do you have a bone or joint problem (e.g. back, knee, or hip) that could be made worse by a change in your physical activity?

Yes ☐ No ☐

Is your doctor currently prescribing drugs (for example, water pills) for your blood pressure or heart condition?

Yes ☐ No ☐

Do you know of any other reason why you should not do physical activity?   Yes ☐ No ☐

If you answered yes to one or more questions
Talk to your doctor by phone or in person BEFORE you start becoming much more active or BEFORE you have a fitness appraisal. Tell your doctor about the PAR-Q and to which questions you answered yes.

► You may be able to do any activity you want as long as you start slowly and build up gradually. Or you may need to restrict your activities to those that are safe for you.

► Talk to your doctor about the kinds of activities you wish to participate in and follow his or her advice.

If you answered no to the PAR-Q questions, you can be reasonably sure that you can:

► Start becoming much more physically active—begin slowly and build up gradually. This is the safest and easiest way.

► Take part in a fitness appraisal—this is an excellent way to determine your basic fitness. It is also highly recommended that you have your blood pressure evaluated. If your reading is higher than 144/94, talk with your doctor before you start becoming much more physically active.

Delay becoming much more active:

► If you are not feeling well because of a temporary illness such as a cold or a fever—wait until you feel better.

► If you are or may be pregnant—talk to your doctor before you start becoming more active.

PLEASE NOTE: If your health changes so that you then answer YES to any of the PAR-Q questions, tell your fitness or health professional. Ask whether you should change your physical activity plan.

Get more active

Doing more in your daily life—walking rather than driving, taking the stairs rather than the elevator—will help burn more calories. Just standing up and moving around is better than sitting. Scientists now think that even if you exercise regularly, too much sitting can negatively affect your health, increasing the risk of type 2 diabetes and heart disease,[6] while just getting up and moving around for two minutes every 20 minutes will help reduce that risk.[7] So on top of your planned exercise, aim to increase the amount of other activity you do during the day and to do it more energetically. Lots of little bits of exercise add up and help to increase your total calorie burn. Being active during the day can burn more calories than a single gym session. For ideas on how to include more physical activity in your daily routine see Appendix F, page 337.

What type of exercise?

For weight loss you need to combine:

▶ Cardiovascular (aerobic) exercise—such as brisk walking, cycling, or swimming, which raises your heart rate and makes you feel warm and slightly out of breath.

▶ Resistance exercise—using light weights, resistance bands, or your own body weight to work your muscles.

Cardiovascular exercise

This type of exercise will help to burn calories and improve your fitness. It lowers your risk of heart disease and some cancers, helps lower blood pressure, improves cholesterol levels, burns off body fat, and is a great antidote to stress. Weight-bearing exercise, when we're on our feet walking and running, is important for maintaining bone density, thereby reducing fracture risk as we age.

> *If I have spent an hour at aerobics burning off 350 calories, the last thing I want to do is replace it all with 350 calories of snacks. Thinking about it, you can eat 350 calories of chocolate or potato chips in just minutes.*
> —Angela, 35

Resistance exercise

This will increase your muscle mass and improve its strength and endurance. More muscle means that your metabolic rate will be higher, so you will burn more calories even at rest and your body will become more toned. Resistance work can also help lower blood pressure and cholesterol and improve insulin sensitivity. It's also important for maintaining strong bones and helping maintain healthy joints, as the muscles supporting those joints strengthen and provide more support. Stronger muscles also mean a lower risk of falls and injuries and will help to improve your balance.

Flexibility exercise

This is another vital, but often overlooked, part of overall fitness. Flexibility tends to decline as you get older, but it's vital for everyday life—you can't do simple things like tie your shoelaces or scrub your back in the bath if you have lost flexibility. Flexibility is specific to each joint or set of joints and refers to the maximum range of movement around that joint. If you stretch regularly as part of your fitness program, you will maintain and improve your flexibility. Maintaining flexibility helps to reduce the risk of injury while you are exercising.

Your exercise targets

In the short term (the first six months), you are aiming to build up to 150 minutes' moderate or 75 minutes' vigorous cardio-vascular exercise per week. Vigorous activity will raise your heart rate higher and burn more calories than moderate exercise. This amount of exercise can feel daunting if you're not used to it, so build up to it gradually. You can break it down into shorter sessions and still receive significant health benefits. You may have heard about recent research suggesting that you only need to exercise at high intensity for a few minutes each week. While this has been shown to have some health benefits, it won't have a major impact on your weight. To ensure that The 2-Day Diet works most effectively you need to exercise for the recommended amount each week.

Moderate exercise Burns 3–5 times as many calories as many being at rest	Vigorous exercise Burns at least six times as calories as being at rest
Walking at 2½–4 mph (4–6.4 kph)	Fast walking (4½ mph/7.2 kph or 4 mph/6.4 kph uphill) or jogging (4 mph/6.4 kph) or quicker
Mowing the lawn	Chopping wood
Badminton	Tennis
Ballroom dancing	High-impact aerobics
Leisurely cycling at 6 mph (9.6 kph)	Faster cycling (10 mph/16 kph)
Recreational swimming at a leisurely pace	Swimming (10 lengths of an 82 ft/25 m pool in 5 minutes—any stroke)

You can break your exercise into five shorter sessions (5 × 30 minutes moderate or 5 × 15 minutes vigorous) or do longer sessions less frequently. (This does not include any warm-up or cool-down exercises.) If you decide on longer sessions, try to exercise three times a week, since some important health benefits (e.g., cholesterol reduction) only last for 48 hours after exercise. You can combine moderate and vigorous exercise and vary your exercise levels from day to day according to your schedule—on a busy day, for example, you may only manage a 15-minute jog, while another day you might have time to swim for an hour.

In the longer term (six months after starting exercising), you should aim to do 300 minutes of moderate or 150 minutes of vigorous exercise a week because this is the level at which the exercise will help you to lose weight, keep it off, and obtain additional health benefits.[8]

As well as your cardiovascular exercise, aim to fit in two to three muscle-strengthening resistance exercise sessions each week and two to three flexibility sessions, to reduce the risk of injury and to stay as mobile as possible. Although this might sound daunting, you can combine the sessions. Stretch by doing a warm-up and cool-down every time you exercise, and add some resistance training to your program a couple of times a week.

On your mark . . .
Think carefully about what you want to achieve—and, more important, what is realistic for you. Exercise should be achievable, enjoyable, and affordable and fit in with your lifestyle and any physical conditions you may have.

Which exercise is best for me?
If you're a complete beginner, you can't go wrong with walking—it's the best free exercise program there is. For anyone with joint or respiratory problems, swimming provides a whole-body workout, although it's not weight bearing and won't help maintain healthy bones. Cycling is another non-weight-bearing

exercise that's good for joints. Recumbent bikes, where your thighs are in a forward position at 90 degrees to your body, are better for people with back or shoulder problems. Running or jogging is a great free activity, but it can strain your knee and hip joints, especially if you run on hard surfaces—you need to wear good-quality running shoes to protect your joints. If you find it hard to stay motivated, exercise classes provide variety and a great social environment and are good for beginners. If you feel too self-conscious to join a class or put on a swimsuit, invest in an exercise DVD or start by borrowing one from the library. Try to find the approach that suits you.

> *Feeling trimmer encourages me to exercise*
> *and makes me more positive.* —Lorna, 53

Wherever you start, the key is to commit yourself. Like you, most regular exercisers have busy lives. The difference is that they make exercise a priority. It takes around three months to form an exercise habit, so schedule it into your life. Look at what you can clear from your calendar, identify any spare time you can use to fit in some activity, and consider dropping some inactivity (like watching TV) to fit your exercise in.

Choose the time of day that suits you best. Exercising early in the day will help to elevate your mood and energy levels for the day. It's important to warm up properly, as your body temperature is lower in the morning, which can increase the risk of injury. When you exercise in the afternoon or evening, you tend to put in more effort since exercise feels easier and your muscles are warm.

Exercising out of doors has added benefits, particularly in the summer months, when exposure to sunshine will increase your production of vitamin D (winter UV light is not strong enough).

Get set . . .

As with your weight loss, setting yourself some short- and longer-term exercise goals gives you a clear idea of what you're aiming for and helps you track your progress.

▶ **Be specific.** Experts agree that successful exercisers are the ones who set specific goals—just deciding to "get fit" or "do more walking" are not specific enough and won't get done. Try to set goals for specific activities with a distance and a time to achieve it in. You might want to set short-term goals, such as being able to walk to the store and back without being out of breath or being able to play a short game of catch with your grandchildren. For the longer term, you will want to aim at something more ambitious, such as setting yourself a 12-week challenge to build up to swim 30 lengths or walk 6 miles (10 km) or even do a 3- or 6-mile (5- or 10-km) charity run.

▶ **Make it achievable.** Be ambitious but realistic. You can always revise your goals if you reach your target very quickly.

▶ **Give yourself deadlines.** Make sure you give yourself a realistic time frame to achieve your goal. You may want to break your goal down into more manageable weekly targets.

▶ **Write yourself a contract.** Write down what you want to achieve and why, how you plan to do it, and how other people can help. Make copies of your contract and pin them up around your home. Think about creating a blog or a Facebook post saying what you are aiming for and how you plan to achieve it. Once others know about your plans, it will make it harder to give up, and you'll get other people on board to encourage you.

▶ **Schedule your exercise.** Book exercise appointments with yourself in your datebook or calendar and stick to them; get up 30 minutes earlier, swap 30 minutes of TV for exercise, or get (or borrow) a dog to walk!

Stay safe

▶ Build up your exercise program slowly to reduce the likelihood of injuries.

▶ Wear loose, comfortable clothing and choose the right footwear with a good arch support—especially if you are walking or running.

▶ Warm up gently before exercising and cool down slowly afterward to help prevent injury and help your body adapt and recover (see below).

▶ Always do your stretches on starting and finishing your training.

▶ Don't overexert yourself; signs of overexertion include nausea, sickness, dizziness, light-headedness, and chest pain.

▶ Don't exercise outside if the weather is too hot or too cold or if you are unwell.

▶ Don't eat a big meal before exercise—wait at least one hour after eating before exercising.

▶ Drink plenty of water.

Warm-up

Preparing your joints for exercise helps to reduce the wear and tear on them. You can do these mobilizing exercises while you march on the spot—to get your heart rate up and prepare your body for activity. Be aware of your posture as you begin to exercise and try to maintain good posture while exercising. Stand tall and slightly draw the stomach muscles toward the spine to engage the abdominal muscles. Looking forward, relax the shoulders down and try to make them straight by drawing the shoulder blades together. Place feet hip-width apart. Knees should not be locked straight but relaxed and have a slight bend. It's important to complete movements in a gentle, smooth manner—not forcing the joints and pushing them beyond the point where it feels uncomfortable. Repeat each mobility exercise six to ten times.

Joint	Mobility exercise	Description
Head/ neck	Neck tilt	Tilt your head, sending the ear toward your left shoulder, then back to the central position, then to your right shoulder.
	Neck turn	Turn your head, looking as far left as you can turn it, then back to the middle, then look as far right as you can.
	Chin retraction	Draw your head straight backward without tilting your chin down, as if you're trying to make a double chin.
Shoulders	Shoulder shrug	Raise your shoulders up toward the ears and then relax back down.
	Shoulder roll	With arms by the sides, roll your shoulders in circles, starting by raising your shoulders toward your ears, then taking them back, down, and around in a circle.
	Arm circles	Progress from the shoulder roll by placing your hands on your shoulders, then making circles as if drawing circles with your elbows. Then extend the arm so that it's straight, and continue the circling. If it feels uncomfortable, try one arm at a time.

Thoracic spine (upper back)	Torso twist	Keeping your hips facing forward, rotate only the upper part of the body, so that your shoulders and head are in line, twisting first left and then right.
Lumbar spine (lower back)	Side bend	Try to remain as straight as possible, as if suspended between two panes of glass. Keep both feet on the floor and tilt your whole body, first to the left and then to the right.
Lumbar spine and hips	Hip circles	Take your hips around in a circle, first clockwise and then counterclockwise.
Knee and hip	Knee to hip	Raise your left leg in front, with the knee bent until it reaches hip height. Repeat with right.
Ankle	Foot point forward and back	Without placing any weight on your leg, point the toes away from your body and then point them back to your body while pushing the heel away.

Pre-exercise stretches

Stretching helps prepare your warmed muscles for further exercise and reduces the risk of injury. Hold each stretch for 10 to 15 seconds on each side.

Calf (gastrocnemius)

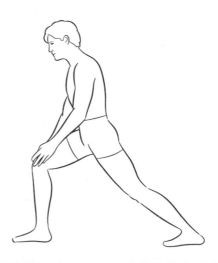

In a standing position, take a step forward and place your right foot out in front, in line with your hips. Your left leg remains outstretched behind you. Lean gently forward, placing your hands on your right knee for support. You should feel the stretch at the top of your left calf. Try to keep your feet facing forward and parallel. Don't let the heel on the left leg that's behind you turn inward.

Back of thigh (hamstring)

In a standing position, take a small step forward with your right leg. Keep this leg straight and outstretched in front of you, while gently bending your left leg (as though you're squatting) and pushing your bottom backward. You should feel this stretch in the top of the back of your leg. You can place your hands on your bent knee for support.

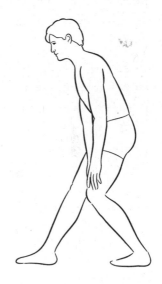

Front of thigh (quadriceps)

Stand near a wall for support. Bring the heel of your right foot back up toward your buttocks. Hold it with one arm (you can use the other to balance yourself). You should feel this stretch down the front of your thigh. If not, gently tilt your pelvis forward until you feel the stretch.

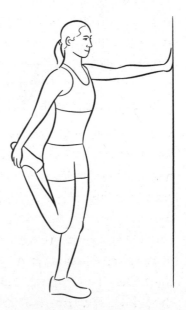

Side (lats and obliques)

In a standing position, with your feet facing forward in line with your hips, place your right hand on your right hip and lift your left arm up along your side and over your head. At the same time, lean to your right. You should feel the stretch from under your arm all the way down the left side of your torso.

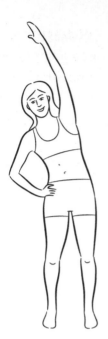

Shoulder

In a standing position, place your right arm across your body, making sure not to lock your elbow. Then, using your left arm, place your hand on your upper right arm and gently pull your right arm in toward your body.

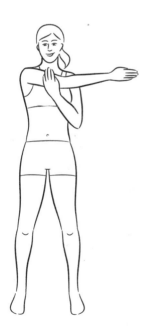

Back of arm (triceps)

In a standing position, raise one arm straight above your head. Bend the elbow so that your hand is reaching down to touch the back of your shoulder. Use the other hand to support the raised arm.

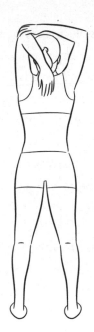

Shoulder (pectorals and deltoid)

Standing side-on to the wall, place your right palm against it. Take one or two steps forward, keeping your palm flat against the wall. Allow your palm to turn so your fingers are pointing backward. Allow your body to twist slightly to the left. You should feel the stretch in your shoulder and across your chest.

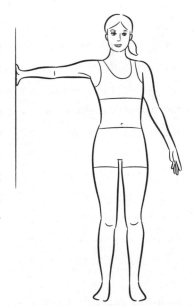

Cool-down

Slow down gradually, over four to six minutes, to help your heart rate and breathing return to normal. If you stop suddenly, without cooling down, it can leave you feeling dizzy, sick, or faint. As you get fitter, your body will respond more readily to changes in physical exertion, and your heart rate will return to normal more quickly. Repeat your warm-up stretches, but this time hold them for up to 60 seconds to help improve your flexibility and prevent stiffness.

Cardiovascular exercise

If you're a complete beginner, walking is, without doubt, the cheapest, easiest, and safest way to get fit. Start gently and aim to walk at a pace that is comfortable for you, but which makes you feel slightly warm and slightly out of breath but still able to talk. Plan a route that is circular, safe, preferably flat, and ideally interesting. Don't worry too much about the distance—as you become fitter, you will be able to walk farther in the same time. Walking is a very safe form of exercise, so you won't necessarily need to warm up unless you're doing morning walks or longer, faster walks.

We've designed a 12-week program so you can build up over the weeks. If the first week feels too easy, start at the level of week three or four. If you're struggling, repeat a week until you're ready to move on. You must complete the full 12 weeks. By your twelfth week you should be doing 150 minutes' moderate exercise—that's about half an hour for five days a week—wherever you were at the start. For your 12-week walking plan, see Appendix G, page 338.

Monitor your cardiovascular progress

It is important to monitor yourself to ensure that you are exercising at the right intensity and that you are exercising safely.

The Talk Test is a simple way to check whether you're working at the right level. You should be a little breathless but still able to hold a conversation. If you're struggling to talk in sentences, you're overdoing it and need to slow down.

The Rate of Perceived Exertion (RPE) is a numerical scale from 1 to 10 (with 1 being the lowest intensity and 10 the highest) that you can use while exercising to gauge how you are feeling and know whether you need to speed up or slow down to be training at the right intensity.

▶ 0 = No exertion at all

▶ 1 = Very, very light exertion

▶ 2 = Very light exertion

▶ 3 = Light exertion

▶ 4 = Moderate exertion

▶ 5 = Somewhat hard (you need to make an effort to maintain a conversation)

▶ 6 = Hard

▶ 7 = Very hard

▶ 8 = Very, very hard

▶ 9 = Extremely hard

▶ 10 = Absolute maximal effort (no conversation is possible, and breathing is very hard)

You'll get the most benefits from exercise when you are working at least at a moderate intensity (4 to 5 on the scale). You should feel slightly warm and be breathing more heavily but still be able to talk. Try to maintain this level for the exercise period—if it gets too easy, pick up the pace. If you are struggling, tone the pace down. Practice using the system while walking before you try it in other exercise situations. As well as keeping you on track, it will help you to monitor your progress—as you get fitter, you may find that you score the same walk or run a 3 instead of a 4.

Resistance exercise

You are aiming to increase your amount of body muscle as well as the endurance and strength of your muscles. For endurance training, you need a lighter weight or smaller resistance and more repetitions. For strength training, you need a heavier weight or greater resistance and fewer repetitions.

We've designed the resistance sessions to work for everyone, whatever their fitness level. Do them two or three times a week to help maintain your muscle mass while you're losing weight. Always do a warm-up and cool-down before and after resistance training.

▶ Keep your movements slow and controlled, both when you contract and relax the muscle.

▶ Focus on your breathing—you should breathe out on exertion and breathe in as you relax the muscle. As with the stretches, avoid holding your breath when you're concentrating on an exercise.

▶ Think about your posture and balance. Stand in front of a mirror to check your posture. Stand tall—imagine a string attached to the top of your head pulling upward—with your shoulders relaxed and down and your weight balanced equally on each foot, with your feet hip-width apart. Good posture will help the important core muscles around your back and stomach area to do their job properly.

▶ These exercises shouldn't hurt or be uncomfortable—if they are, stop!

▶ Avoid locking your elbows or knees straight or over-extending joints.

▶ Familiarize yourself with the jargon. Exercise programs often refer to "sets" and "reps" (repetitions), so "one set of 10 reps" for a bicep curl would be 10 repetitions of a bicep curl, and two sets of 10 reps would be 10 repetitions, a pause or rest, and then another 10 repetitions.

You can do repetitive resistance exercises using free weights (dumbbells), resistance bands, the weight of your own body, inflatable exercise balls, or one of the many different exercise gadgets on the market. Free weights don't have to cost you a penny. Water weighs 1 g per ml, so if you fill a 500 ml (16.9 fl oz) plastic water bottle, your handmade weight will be 500 g (1 lb 1 oz). To make heavier weights, fill bottles with sand. Once you start needing heavier weights, you might want to think about buying a set. Latex resistance bands come in a variety of colors, which refer to their thickness. The thicker they are, the tougher they are to stretch and the more resistance they produce. They can be used with most exercises: for example, to do bicep curls, place the resistance band on the floor and position your foot in the middle of the band. Pick up an end of the band in either hand, making sure you have a good grip. You can then use the resistance of the band to do your bicep curls. Don't wrap the band around your hand and cut off the blood flow. If you're using your own body weight for a resistance exercise—for example for a push-up—make sure you start with the easiest position before you progress over time: for example, start by pressing from all fours and progress to full-on toes push-ups.

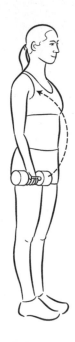

Bicep curls

Active muscles: Biceps (front of arm)

Description: Stand with your feet shoulder-width apart and your arms down by your sides, palms facing forward. With a light weight in your right hand, bring the weight up toward the shoulder. Bend the elbow, but keep it by your side. Switch arms and repeat.

Progression: 1. Try doing both arms together.
　　　　　　　 2. Increase the weight.

Triceps extension

Active muscles: Triceps (back of arm)

Description: Lying on the floor on your back with a light weight in your right hand, raise it straight above your head, then gently bending your elbow, lower the weight to the side of your head. Switch arms and repeat.

Progression: 1. Try doing both arms together.
　　　　　　　 2. Increase the weight.
　　　　　　　 3. Do the exercise standing up, allowing the arm and weight to go behind the head.

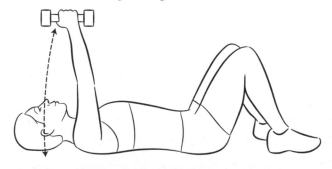

Push-ups

Active muscles: Chest (pectoral muscles)

Description: Kneeling on all fours, with your hands flat on the floor, shoulder-width apart, lift your feet off the floor so that the weight is now on your knees and arms. Slowly bend your elbows, keeping your back straight, taking your nose to the ground.

Progression: 1. Extend your legs, going up onto your toes, spreading your legs apart, and repeat.

                2. Extend your legs, going up onto your toes and keep your feet together.

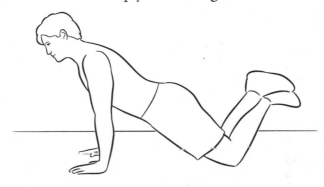

Plank

Active muscles: Abdominals

Description: Lying on your front with your palms and all of your lower arm in contact with the floor, think of yourself from neck to toes as one long, rigid piece of wood. Raise yourself up (the palm and lower arm stay in contact with the floor), and you're on your toes in a position similar to a push-up but much closer to the floor. Hold this straight, horizontal plank position. Be very careful if you suffer from lower-back problems. Try not to cave in and let your stomach fall to the floor. If the plank feels too intense, relax to the floor and try an easier version on all fours. Progress by moving your knee position farther back, until your legs are straight as below.

Progression: 1. While you are in the plank position, raise one
leg 2.5 cm (1 in) off the ground, hold for two
seconds, and switch legs.

2. Rotate to the side so that your elbow, shoulder, and head are in a line.

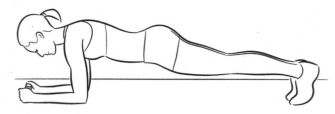

Single-arm row

Active muscles: Back and biceps

Description: Stand with your feet shoulder-width apart, legs
and back straight. Lean forward, holding a weight in one hand,
and, arm extended, pull the weight back toward you, bending
the elbow. Repeat with the other arm.

Progression: 1. Exercise both arms together.

2. Increase weight.

3. Lean over farther (make sure your back is
straight).

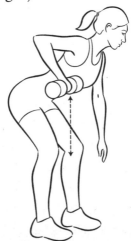

Squats

Active muscles: Thighs and buttocks (hamstrings, quadriceps, and gluteal muscles)

Description: Stand with your feet slightly wider than hip-width apart, with both feet facing forward. Slowly push your buttocks backward, and then, keeping a straight back, shoulders and your head up, bend at the knees in a sitting motion.

Progression: 1. Raise your arms up straight as you squat.

                 2. Try the same thing, but with small weights.

                 3. Try while doing arm weights (e.g., bicep curls).

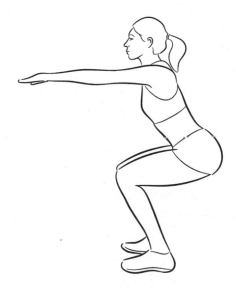

Home circuit class

For a complete workout, combine cardiovascular, resistance, and flexibility training, and make yourself a home circuit using five or six of the above resistance exercises. Alternate between leg and arm exercises to prevent fatigue, and add marching, side-stepping, or skipping in between each strengthening exercise to raise your heart rate. Start with low, or no, weights and slowly increase as you progress. Gradually add more exercises to your circuit and increase the number of repetitions and sets that you do. Cool down and stretch to complete your workout. The exercises that you can do with weights are marked * in the table.

I have enjoyed getting into clothes that haven't fitted for a long time, and I'm really feeling the benefits of increased fitness from exercise. —Sam, 29

Exercise	Week 1	Week 4	Week 8
Bicep curls*	1 set x 10 reps	2 sets x 10 reps	3 sets x 10 reps
Triceps extensions*	1 set x 10 reps	2 sets x 10 reps	3 sets x 10 reps
Push-ups	1 set x 10 reps	2 sets x 10 reps	3 sets x 10 reps
Plank	2 sets 20-second holds	2 sets 30-second holds	3 sets 40-second holds
Single-arm row	1 set x 10 reps	2 sets x 10 reps	3 sets x 10 reps
Squat	1 set x 10 reps	2 sets x 10 reps	3 sets x 10 reps

After the first 12 weeks . . .

You can continue with the same exercise program for the next three months, to give your body time to adapt before you step things up to aim for 300 minutes of moderate or 150 minutes' vigorous cardiovascular exercise a week. If you feel ready to do more before the end of the three months, go for it! Remember that you don't have to stick with the same exercise classes or activity, but you should keep doing the same amount of exercise, at the same level of intensity.

How to stay motivated

Vary your routine

Change what you do every six to eight weeks to avoid getting bored and reaching a plateau in your fitness. If you keep doing the same exercise, your body will adapt to it so it is no longer challenging and your fitness won't improve. For example, if you're walking, include some hills or find a new route; if you are swimming, vary your strokes or add a completely different type of exercise to your weekly schedule. If you're a gym member, ask your trainer to design you a new program every three months.

Find a new challenge

Learning a new skill is always empowering, so if you are feeling more body-confident now, why not learn to dance? Ballroom dancing is not just for the celebrities. Alternatively, why not revisit a sport you used to play—perhaps one you loved in your school days? Perhaps you used to play tennis but stopped? Find a local club for new people to play with.

Measure yourself

Waist, hips, and bust are the most obvious parts of the body to measure, but you might want to keep track of your upper-arm or thigh measurements. Measure your waist to see whether you're losing abdominal fat (see page 34).

Record the changes

The camera never lies, so why not keep "before" and "after" photos pinned up on your fridge to help keep you on track and focused on your exercise regime. Visible evidence of the way your body is changing will encourage you to persevere.

Just do a little

When you feel pushed for time or really demotivated, just try to do 10 minutes of activity. You're getting some health benefits, and you might find that by committing to doing 10 minutes of exercise, you end up doing more.

Be flexible

If your exercise bike breaks, don't give up until it's fixed: try something different. If you have less time one week to fit in your exercise sessions, try to exercise harder for less time. Life tends to throw lots of things at us, and we can't let it derail our good intentions.

Monitor your workouts

If you feel the frequency of your workouts might be slipping, use apps or a simple journal to monitor yourself and to remind you to exercise.

Sign up

Try entering a sponsored swim, run, or bike ride. Alternatively, sponsor yourself and give a donation to charity when you have achieved a personal fitness goal.

Adapt your exercise program

If you know you're heading toward a busy month, or if you feel your time commitment to exercise is wavering, think about changing your approach and focus on intensity rather than frequency. If you've been exercising at a moderate level, increase the intensity of your workout to a vigorous level and decrease the frequency of your workouts. This way, you're meeting the recommended exercise guidelines in literally half the time.

Reward yourself

Set yourself mini goals every couple of weeks—to walk farther, faster; add five minutes to your routine—and give yourself a reward (that's not food or alcohol) when you achieve your goal.

Your questions answered

How will I know if I'm getting fitter?

Take your resting pulse rate. Sit down for five minutes (10 if you've been active). Then place two fingers on the inside of your wrist and count the number of pulse beats in a minute. Do this weekly—as you get fitter, your pulse rate will get slower.

Do a simple walking/running test. Walk or run a mile. Time how long it takes you, measure your pulse at the end, and score your RPE (see page 135). Repeat the test after 12 weeks.

Will exercise make me hungry?

We all react differently to increasing our activity levels—half of us naturally eat more; the other half either eat less or roughly the same amount.[9] As you step up your exercise, monitor your eating and make sure you don't reward yourself or "compensate" for exercise done by having larger servings or "treats" of high-sugar, high-fat foods.

Exercise is actually well known for helping to regulate your appetite, and doing some activity on restricted days could help to distract you and keep you from getting bored, especially in the evenings, when you might be tempted to break your diet.

Should I have a sports drink to keep my energy levels up?

Staying well hydrated while exercising is vital for your energy levels and your overall health, but water is the best thing to drink. A 17½ fl oz (500 ml) sports drink contains between 150 and 350 calories, most of it sugar. Ignore the marketing hype—unless you're an elite athlete in training, you're unlikely to need anything more than water.

How many calories will I burn?

It's tempting to think that if you're exercising, you can eat what you like—in fact, as you can see below, it takes a lot of exercise to burn off even a small amount of food. The number of calories burned has been estimated for a woman weighing 154 lb (70 kg).[10] If you are heavier than this, you will burn off slightly more calories during each activity; if you are lighter, you will burn off slightly fewer.

Half an hour of . . .	Calories burned by a 154 lb (70 kg) woman	Examples of food burned off
Vacuuming	115	10 fl oz (300 ml) of orange juice 4 thin mint fondant-filled chocolates 3 wrapped chocolates
Gardening: moderate effort	122	A ¾ oz (25 g) bag of potato chips 8 oz bottle orange-carrot juice A 4 oz (125 g) whole-milk yogurt
Walking 3.5 mph (5.6 kph)	150	A 1½ oz (40 g) fondant-filled chocolate egg 12 oz beer 1¼ oz (35 g) cheddar cheese
Aerobics: low impact	175	2 chocolate graham crackers A 6 fl oz (175 ml) glass of wine A 2 oz (60 g) scoop premium ice cream
Swimming: breaststroke, light recreational	185	A small bottle (13 fl oz/380 ml) of energy drink 3 plain graham crackers A 1 oz (30 g) bag of potato chips

Half an hour of ...	Calories burned by a 154 lb (70 kg) woman	Examples of food burned off
Cycling 9 mph (14.5 kph)	203	Half a cheese sandwich A roll of hard candy A large latte coffee
Aerobics: high impact	255	A 8½ fl oz (250 ml) glass of wine A 15½ fl oz (440 ml) can beer 1¾ oz (50 g) of milk chocolate
Jogging 5 mph (8 kph)	290	7 oz (200 g) chicken chow mein (takeout) 17½ fl oz (500 ml) cola Half a double burger (3½ oz/108 g) (fast-food outlet)
Running 7 mph (11 kph)	384	7 oz (200 g) egg fried rice (takeout) 4 oz (117 g) medium serving French fries A fast-food medium strawberry milk shake

Can I spot-reduce problem areas like my bottom and waist?

Although there's no evidence that you can spot-reduce fat by spending a lot of time exercising specific areas, what does seem clear is that you tend to lose fat more quickly from some areas of the body than others when you lose weight and do exercise. Getting your recommended 150–300 minutes of moderate cardiovascular exercise—doing things like brisk walking or jogging—can boost the loss of unhealthy intra-abdominal fat, which should both improve your health and reduce your waist measurement.[11] And although we still don't have conclusive evidence, we think that the two strict days of dieting each week with The 2-Day Diet could have a greater impact on abdominal fat. Exercise will also tone muscles, helping you to feel more toned in areas such as your buttocks, thighs, and abdomen.

Can I exercise on restricted days of the diet?

Lots of people think that because they are limiting calories, and particularly carbs, they won't have the energy to exercise on the restricted two days of The 2-Day Diet. In fact, we found that this wasn't the case. Our Dieters were just as likely to exercise on the two restricted as on the five unrestricted days, and the calorie and carbohydrate restrictions didn't seem to reduce their ability to exercise or increase their levels of fatigue. Some of the Dieters actually recorded 60 minutes of vigorous activity and as much as four hours of moderate activity on the restricted days of the diet. Other research bears out the fact that your exercise capacity and tolerance shouldn't dip on restricted days[12]—in fact, one study suggested that if you are doing a low-carb, low-calorie diet, you might burn more fat while exercising than if you were following a high-carb, low-cal diet. Make sure you stay well hydrated and get your sodium, potassium, and permitted 50 g of carbohydrates in your dairy, fruit, and vegetable allowance.

If you are normally a vigorous exerciser and are struggling with this on your two restricted days of The 2-Day Diet, we recommend replacing vigorous with moderate activity and saving the vigorous workouts for your unrestricted days.

Is it better to exercise before breakfast or when I haven't eaten for a while, or to exercise after meals?

When you exercise, your body takes energy from carbohydrates, or if they're not available, from burning your fat stores. A question that has intrigued sports scientists is whether exercizing when you haven't eaten for a while—in other words, when there is no available carbohydrate energy—can boost the amount of fat you burn. A recent study suggests that this may be the case. In a very carefully controlled experiment, researchers in Glasgow asked 10 overweight and normally sedentary men to walk for an hour either immediately before or immediately after a 450-calorie breakfast. They then monitored how much fat was burned off during the exercise and for eight and a half hours afterward. Although both exercise sessions burned fat, the men who exercised before breakfast burned 40 percent more fat than those who walked after eating.[13] So although exercising at any time will help with your weight loss, you may get an extra boost from doing it before, rather than soon after, meals.

Using a pedometer

A pedometer is a great way to track your walking progress or to measure how much more activity you're clocking up in a normal day. We should all be aiming for between 7,000 and 11,000 steps per day, and at least 3,000 should be done at a brisk pace.

Pedometers work by sensing the force your body generates when you take a step. You clip them onto your waistband, and they add up your steps as you get on with your life. Because they sense force, be aware that they can also record nonwalking activities such as going over a speed bump when driving! Avoid the cheapest machines, which can be unreliable, and go for a midrange model. Make sure your pedometer does not slip or turn during walking, or it may not record correctly.

To check that a new pedometer is measuring accurately, walk 50 steps. If it is not correct, ensure that it is vertical on your hip and move it around until you find a place where it gives you an accurate count. Some pedometers are worn as watches or carried in a pocket, but again, try to test them for accuracy. Some pedometers provide you with an estimate of calories burned and distance covered. It is important to remember that these estimates are not tailored to you and so are not a reliable measure. If you want to measure calories burned, look for a pedometer that allows you to input your weight, height, gender, and stride length if you want to know the distance you are covering. Some companies have designed pedometers that can link to your phone or MP3 player (sometimes worn as an armband or on shoes), and some can be linked to your computer so you can download your daily steps and track your progress.

Dealing with problems

Aching muscles

Don't be surprised if your muscles protest a bit at first—you'll find you will probably ache most 48 hours after exercising! It will get better. Doing a proper warm-up and cool-down is thought to decrease the risk of injury, especially if you are not used to exercise.

Dehydration

Stay hydrated. Drink water rather than sports drinks, which tend to be loaded with sugar and calories. If you've had a particularly sweaty workout, try a small glass of fat-free milk to replenish your electrolyte and sugar levels.

Joint pain

Muscle-strengthening exercises, Pilates, or yoga will help strengthen muscles supporting your joints and should help with knee and hip pain, but if you have achy joints, you should see your GP. Although the evidence is limited, you might want to try glucosamine and/or chondroitin sulfate. There's some evidence that a daily 1,500 mg glucosamine supplement can provide modest pain relief for some people. Check with your GP before taking any health dietary supplement.

Fatigue

Exercise can make you feel a little tired, but if you need to sit down for more than 30 minutes afterward, you're overdoing it, and you need to slow down. Try reducing the frequency and the intensity of the exercise and see how you feel next time.

Injury

If you build up exercise gradually at your own pace, you shouldn't get injured, but if you do, see your GP and physiotherapist and take their advice about how quickly to return to exercising. Rehabilitation exercise, such as swimming (after receiving the okay from your GP), is an easy and supportive form of exercise to get you back into the swing of things.

Should I buy a heart rate monitor?

You don't need to buy one, but if you like the idea of having a gadget that can tell you whether you are working hard enough and help monitor your progress, you might want to invest in a basic monitor (priced around $25 to $40), and you can upgrade as you progress. Some are like watches, which take your thumb pulse when placed on the screen; others use separate chest straps that register and transmit your heart rate to a watch every few seconds. You can also download a heart rate monitor as an app to your mobile phone. Using heart rate zones allows you to

exercise safely at different intensities. Your maximum heart rate
(in beats per minute) is 220 minus your age, so if you are 40, it will
be 180 beats per minute.

The different heart rate zones, which work in percentages of
your maximum heart rate, are:

- Moderate exercise = 50 to 70%
  50–60% of maximum heart rate = Moderate Aerobic Zone
  60–70% of maximum heart rate = Aerobic Weight
  Management Zone

- Vigorous exercise = 70 to 85%
  70–80% of maximum heart rate = Aerobic Fitness Zone
  80–90% of maximum heart rate = Peak Aerobic Performance
  Zone

Exercising at a heart rate between 80% and 90% of maximum
heart rate is suitable only for trained individuals.

Summary

▶ Regular exercise will enhance the benefits of The 2-Day Diet
by burning calories and maintaining calorie-burning muscle.
It also helps protect against heart disease, type 2 diabetes,
and many cancers and will boost your mood and energy
levels.

▶ Before starting an exercise program, make sure that you are
fit enough. If in doubt, see your GP.

▶ To benefit your health you need to do 150 minutes of
moderate or 75 minutes of vigorous exercise each week. For

weight loss and added health benefits, you need to build up to 300 minutes of moderate or 150 minutes of vigorous exercise each week.

▶ Aim to do strengthening exercises 2–3 times per week.

▶ Try to do exercises that will improve your flexibility 2 times per week.

▶ It's important to combine cardiovascular exercise with resistance exercises to strengthen your muscles and stretching to improve flexibility.

▶ You can break exercise into smaller or longer chunks and do it every day or less frequently, but ideally you should exercise at least once every two days.

▶ Ensure that you warm up and cool down properly each time you exercise, to help avoid injury.

▶ Once you get into the exercise habit, set yourself new goals and vary your routine to avoid becoming bored.

7

how to
stay slim

Congratulations! If you are reading this chapter, you have probably reached your weight-loss goal with The 2-Day Diet and are ready to move into the next phase: keeping the pounds off and maintaining your fantastic new look and weight. We know that it's taken huge commitment and a lot of hard work to get to this point, and you need to give yourself a huge pat on the back for your amazing achievement.

But let's pause here—your work is not yet done! The big temptation for any dieter who has achieved a goal weight is to accept the praise, heave a huge sigh of relief that the diet is over, and go back to eating the way he or she did before starting the diet. And some of you reading this will have been there already—possibly several times—and will know how devastating it feels when you see the weight starting to creep back on.

But don't worry! This chapter will give you the tools you need to make sure that this doesn't happen again. You haven't done all this hard work only to go back to where you started. The vital thing to recognize is that having reached your weight-loss goal is not the end, but an important transition time. Like losing weight, *maintaining* the weight you have achieved will take commitment, vigilance, and perseverance. It can be just as much of a challenge as getting the weight off in the first place, but this time you are able to build on your success and use the skills you have acquired along the way to capitalize on the way you have retrained your eating and your exercise habits.

> *My lapses almost always come when I drink alcohol—for example, after a few glasses of wine on a Friday night. I do well all week, then after a drink I tend to eat more. But now that I know this, I've pretty much cut it out.*
> —Rose, 52

How your body is different

Big changes have taken place in your body since you started The 2-Day Diet. You now weigh less, so your body needs fewer calories for its basic metabolism, upkeep, and movement than it did before you started dieting. If you think of this as being like the difference between walking around as you are now and then with a backpack stuffed with the weight you have lost, you can appreciate why you needed more energy and calories. Losing weight with any diet also means that many hormones in your body will change, including hormones that increase your appetite and stop you from feeling full as quickly.[1] Dieting probably also means that your muscles will have become more efficient and need less energy to function. While this is good news for your muscles, it means that you could now need up to 15 percent fewer calories than someone of the same weight who hasn't dieted.

The bottom line is that having lost your weight, you now need to eat around 400 to 600 fewer calories each day than you did before you started dieting, and you must keep exercising to help burn off calories and offset the changes in your metabolism.[2] If you go back to your previous lifestyle, you will regain the weight at least as quickly as you lost it.

While all this sounds daunting, we know from our own research that 2-Day Dieters can and do succeed in keeping the weight off. Our first 2-Day Diet study followed up our 2-Day Dieters for 12–15 months. This group had lost around 21 lb (9.5 kg), going on average from 179 lb (81 kg) to 159 lb (72 kg) on The 2-Day Diet. They then switched to one restricted day per week to maintain weight loss. After six to nine months of this 1-Day Maintenance Diet, they weighed, on average, 164 lb (74.3 kg)—so had kept off 14 lb (6.4 kg).

Crucially for their health, one restricted day per week had maintained the beneficial reductions in their blood pressure, cholesterol, and insulin. Normally, when you stop following a standard calorie-controlled diet, you revert to eating your full calorie requirements on a daily basis. This is when some of the health benefits you've gained from losing weight, particularly the drop in insulin, blood pressure, and cholesterol, often start to drift upward.

How to keep the weight off

So, to maintain your weight loss, we recommend simply switching to The 1-Day Maintenance Diet as part of our weight maintenance plan. This plan has been designed in the knowledge that weight maintenance is a new challenge that requires you to keep your calorie intake down and exercise levels up. It requires you to build on the skills you have used for weight loss but requires a different way of thinking. The next section highlights the dietary guidelines for the one restricted day and six unrestricted Mediterranean diet days.

This chapter aims to give you the strategies you need to make sure the weight stays off for good.

It's harder to follow the diet when you are out in restaurants or at people's houses when they have cooked for you. You have to make sure you tell them in advance.
—Diana, 49

The 1-Day Maintenance Diet

The 1-Day Maintenance Diet is based on The 2-Day Diet, but instead of two restricted days each week, you now only have to do one. For the rest of the week (the other six days), we advise you to eat the healthy Mediterranean diet you have followed with The 2-Day Diet (see page 70). Like The 2-Day Diet, you should not have to count calories or weigh food for your 1-Day Maintenance Diet but, as before, make sure that you are keeping within the recommended amounts.

Once again, it's important that on your one restricted day you meet the minimum recommended servings for protein, fruit, vegetables, and dairy foods and don't exceed the maximum recommendations for protein and fats. On the six unrestricted days of The 1-Day Maintenance Diet, make sure that you get enough protein, fruit, and vegetables, but keep within the maximum amounts. Don't forget, you will need to check the Diet in the calculators in Appendix D (see pages 327–335), which tells you the number of servings you can eat on these days for your new lower weight. The Diet has been calculated to account for the fact that you are a successful Dieter and has assumed that your weight has dropped and that therefore your energy requirements are likely to have lowered since you first started The 2-Day Diet.

You may recall that after your two restricted days on The 2-Day Diet your weight dropped, partly as a result of losing water. You will also lose water after your one restricted day on The 1-Day Maintenance Diet, so when you weigh yourself, remember to do it just before and not during or immediately after your restricted day.

Adjust your thinking

As well as following a different diet plan, you need to adjust your mental approach to put you in the right frame of mind for keeping the weight off permanently.

In some ways, starting a new diet is the easiest part of weight loss. It's new, you're full of hope for the future, and you hopefully have the support and encouragement of the people around you who are willing you to succeed. And when you do succeed and the weight comes off, your efforts are constantly rewarded by the compliments you receive about how good you look and by the fact that, at long last, you can start to wear the clothes you like and do the things you enjoy.

Weight maintenance is a completely different ball game. You don't have the excitement of a new challenge, and no one is going to marvel and congratulate you about the fact that you are managing to keep the weight off (although they should, because it's a great achievement!). Your challenge now is to make weight control a way of life, using the expertise you've gained from mastering The 2-Day Diet.

> *The times I've not stuck to it have been when I was busy with work, rushing between meetings. It's difficult to control your environment, as you are obliged to take whatever's available—I have had to plan for that.*
> —Theresa, 43

Key tips for maintaining your weight loss

1. Monitor yourself

Keeping a close eye on your weight is a key part of keeping the weight off. If you spot early signs of weight gain, you can act quickly and reverse the trend. Weigh yourself weekly, just as you have done throughout The 2-Day Diet, and keep an eye on how your clothes fit—a garment becoming a bit tight could indicate that you are putting on a few pounds. Don't be tempted to "cheat" by always wearing loose clothing, such as sweatpants, as you're unlikely to notice any change—more snugly fitting clothes are better indicators. If you notice your clothes becoming tighter, weigh yourself. Weight can fluctuate by 2–4½ lb (1–2 kg), but if your weight increases by more than 4½ lb (2 kg) or by 3 percent of your total weight, this is an alarm bell ringing to tell you to get back on track with your diet and exercise plan.

2. Stay motivated

Revisit your original reasons for wanting to lose weight and remind yourself of how far you have come. You set yourself goals at the start of The 2-Day Diet, and it's a really good idea to also set yourself clear targets for keeping the weight off. You might want to keep the weight off for a forthcoming event such as a wedding, a party, or a holiday.

We have already mentioned how you can use "before" dieting photos to motivate yourself to stay on track when losing weight. You can also use "before" and "after" dieting photos to remind yourself what you have achieved with all your hard work and use these as an incentive for keeping the weight off. Clothes that you can now get into, which you could not before starting to diet, are also a great reminder of how far you have come.

Rewards for achieving your goals—and for sticking with your eating and exercise plan—are even more important when it comes to weight maintenance than for losing weight, as you won't have the immediate thrill of seeing the weight coming off. Plan a treat for yourself at the end of each month that you have kept your weight off. In fact, given how challenging it can be, you should probably reward yourself *more* for weight maintenance than you did for weight loss.

3. Set up your support systems

As well as rewarding yourself, we know there is nothing quite as motivating as receiving positive comments and support from the people around you. This may not automatically happen, and so you may need to ask your nearest and dearest for their help. Ask the people who supported you when you were trying to lose weight to carry on with their encouragement as you work at keeping it off. Explain to them that this is an important time for you, with its own challenges. Their support is required to help you keep to your diet plan of one restricted day per week and an unrestricted Mediterranean diet for six days per week, plus your regular exercise plan. Having people to acknowledge your achievements in keeping the weight off is every bit as important as their support for losing weight has been over the months of the diet.

4. Be prepared

The experience of doing The 2-Day Diet will have made you aware of the danger times, which can divert you from your good intentions with eating and exercise. We talked about this in chapters 2 and 5 (see pages 38 and 94), and it might be worth going back to your original list to remind yourself of the strategies that work for you when it comes to fending off temptation or dealing with difficult situations. Use the stress management strategies to overcome the trap of comfort eating, and plan ahead for social situations. You might decide to allow yourself to eat more freely when it comes to particular social events but compensate by eating less in the days before and afterward. If there are occasions when you feel that you have lapsed, don't give up; instead, learn from them to enable you to cope better the next time around.

There can also be longer-term issues that can interfere with weight maintenance. For example, a very busy spell at work when you are stuck in the office until late at night, home improvements that leave you unable to use your kitchen, and periods when you are working away from home and sleeping and eating in hotels can all hamper healthy eating and exercise routines. The good thing is that you can usually see these things looming on the horizon and can plan around them.

If I do lapse I try to get straight back on track
—I may cut back on something else to balance out
"the transgression." —Heather, 57

CASE STUDY: Annabell

Annabell's story shows just what it's possible to achieve. When Annabell, 35, started our first 2-Day Diet, she had a BMI of 38 and weighed almost 203 lb (92 kg). After 15 months on The 2-Day Diet, she had lost nearly 49 lb (22 kg), and five years later, she has maintained that weight loss.

"I had tried low-calorie diets before, and I'd tried just eating less, but although I always lost a few pounds, I quickly got fed up and stopped. The 2-Day Diet worked for me because it was structured. I found the two restricted days of The 2-Day Diet easy because the rules were so clear, and once I reached my goal weight I did The 1-Day Maintenance Diet. I weigh myself once a week, but I can tell by my clothes if I'm gaining weight. I often do one day per week to keep me in check, but I usually gain about 4 lb (1.8 kg) when I go on vacation. Now I just go back onto two days per week of dieting when I get home, and it comes back off. Eating like this has become a way of life, and I'm still getting positive feedback from family and friends. When I started The 2-Day Diet, I was out of breath just walking up stairs; now I regularly do 90-minute brisk walks, play badminton, and go to Zumba. It's changed me: I'm more confident, I'm happier, I can wear skirts for the first time in years, and I have so much more energy to do things with my daughter."

5. Watch for portion creep

By the time they completed The 2-Day Diet, most of our Dieters had a more realistic idea about the size of a healthy serving of food, but it's still important to keep track of your serving sizes. We're not suggesting that you become obsessive and weigh all of your food, but it's surprisingly easy for servings to get bigger without really noticing it. It helps to use the simple household measures we describe to check your servings. For example, don't just pour out the cereal, rice, or pasta; use spoons or a small cup (not a big mug!). It might also help to use smaller plates and bowls and small cutlery. At the end of the day, add up the number of food servings you have had against the recommended amounts for the Diet, using the progress charts at www.the2daydietbook.com.

6. Are you active enough?

Once you reach the maintenance stage, you need to be aiming to do 300 minutes' moderate, or 150 minutes' vigorous, exercise spread over the week (see chapter 6). Again, it can be easy to let this slip, so monitor what you do. All the evidence suggests that successful maintainers keep a close eye on their activity levels as well as their weight. You can do a quick mental tally of how active you have been at the end of each day. Write it in a journal or use an online tool. Don't forget that as you get lighter and fitter, you will find exercise easier. Although this is great, it does also mean that you won't use as many calories when you exercise as when you first started out. This is why, as you lose weight, you need to keep challenging your body with more demanding workouts.

When I go out for meals, I simply have reduced servings to enable me to stick to the Diet, as I am never very sure how the food was prepared. —Alicia, 47

7. Keep it varied

Some of us love routine, but if you feel you are stuck in a rut with your diet and exercise, shake things up. Try different foods, and experiment with some of the other recipes in this book (see chapters 9 and 10), not just the four or five favorites you have done so far. Set yourself some different exercise goals, adapt your routine, introduce a different activity into your weekly routine, or take up a new challenge, such as a half marathon or a charity bike ride.

CASE STUDY: Jane

Jane, 51, has always struggled with her weight. In fact, she took part in three previous weight-loss studies at the Genesis Breast Cancer Prevention Centre, and although she was really successful and lost 28–42 lb (12–19 kg) each time, she also put all the weight back on—and sometimes more—once within just five months of reaching her goal weight. But following The 2-Day Diet has been a very different story: weighing in at the beginning of the Diet at just over 245 lb (111 kg), Jane managed to lose 42 lb (19 kg) within seven months; even more impressive, two and a half years later, she has maintained her weight loss and is thrilled with her success.

"I liked The 2-Day Diet right from the beginning because I was able to be really strict with myself on my two restricted diet days, and although I was careful during the other days, I didn't feel that I was dieting because it was so different. I lost a lot of weight at first, and then it slowed down, but I then joined a gym, which gave me another spurt.

"When I relaxed and didn't do my one day of maintenance each week, I immediately felt the weight going back on, so now I know that to keep the weight off, this needs to be a way of life. But because it's only one day, I find it easy to do—everyone can be 'good' one day a week! It doesn't really impact on my lifestyle, and I can adjust it to suit times like vacations and Christmas. The one time when I struggle is when I am unhappy—then I still crave comfort food. I suppose the answer is to be happy all the time!"

8. Get peer support from other maintainers

It can be enormously helpful to have regular contact with other people who are also trying to keep the weight off. To help you keep on track with your weight maintenance, as well as your dieting, find us on Facebook, where you can get support and ideas from other maintainers.

What happens if my weight creeps back up again?

If you start to notice your weight is increasing, keep a close eye on it. Weight can vary from day to day by as much as 2–4 lb (1–1.8 kg), but if you notice a gradual increase over three or four weeks, then you need to take action straight away. It's relatively easy to shed a few extra pounds, but when that turns into 7 lb (3 kg), it becomes much more difficult. If the weight gain is literally just a pound or two (0.5–1 kg) and you want to get rid of it, check and adjust your diet over the next few weeks and increase your exercise. If you have regained more than this, you should go back on The 2-Day Diet for a few weeks, until you have lost the regained weight—and then go immediately back to The 1-Day Maintenance Diet.

Have you reached your goal, or are you stuck?

If you have achieved the weight you were aiming for or are happy with the amount that you have lost, then follow The 1-Day Maintenance Diet. However, if you feel that you are stuck at a particular weight and unable to move on, and you're reading this chapter because you feel like giving up on your weight-loss goal . . . whatever you do—don't! Although we expect your rate of weight loss to gradually decrease over six to eight months, it shouldn't grind to a halt. In fact, several studies of Dieters under controlled conditions have found that although the majority of weight loss does happen in the first six to eight months, your weight should continue to gradually drop over three years—and then it will reach a plateau. So you would lose half of the total weight you lose in the first year and the second half in the following two years.[3]

If your weight loss has ground to a halt, then it's time to go back to basics. The reduction in your metabolic rate could be an important factor in slowing down your weight loss, but it shouldn't stop it altogether. The main reason why weight loss reaches a plateau is because, understandably, people become less vigilant about their diet and exercise regime over time without even realizing it's happening. It may be a few weeks since you stopped being as rigorous about your diet and exercise as you were, but you assumed it was okay because you kept losing weight until you eventually plateaued. Check that you really are sticking to the eating and exercise plans as carefully as you were in week one of your 2-Day Diet. If you are not following these plans to the letter, as you were when you started the Diet, go back to those chapters (see pages 44 and 116) and remind yourself of the rules. To get back on track, it may help to keep a diet and exercise journal to record your eating and activity levels.

CASE STUDY: Linda

Linda, 31, started to gain weight in her mid-20s and was 158 lb (71.6 kg) by the time she started The 2-Day Diet. "I had always been active and a healthy weight, but a combination of university and a love for triple chocolate muffins meant that I went from a size 8 to a size 12, and my weight shot up from 137 lb (62 kg) to a not-so-healthy 168 lb (76 kg). I lost a bit of weight over the next few years, but I was still around 150 lb (68 kg), and although I had a relatively healthy diet, my serving sizes were way out of control and I did no exercise. After one Christmas, when my weight had gone up to 157 lb (71.2 kg) and my mother had developed severe complications of diabetes, I realized that I had to do something about my weight or I would make myself ill.

"I'd started exercising more, but it usually left me really hungry and my weight loss was slow, probably because I was overeating. I decided on The 2-Day Diet because I don't have the willpower for seven days a week. I'm vegetarian, so the low-carb days made me look carefully at what I was eating and see where there were imbalances.

"With the added incentive of my wedding, I decided that 2012 was a sink-or-swim year. The diet was quite hard at first, and I was hungry by Day Two, but the two days left me feeling lighter and somehow 'cleaner' on the inside. A few weeks into it, I didn't notice the hunger anymore, but the thing I really liked was that I could choose which two consecutive days to do. So if we had planned a meal out, I'd switch my days so I wasn't restricting myself that day. Crucially, I didn't feel as though I was missing out. Only restricting myself for two days also meant that I had the energy to exercise on the other days—something I don't think I could have stuck to if the restriction had been continuous.

"My weight loss has been gradual, but maintained. You have to spend the first couple of weeks getting used to the Diet, but the longer you stick with it—the easier it gets. And I finally understand serving sizes. Best of all I was a size 8 for my wedding!"

Summary

▶ Congratulate yourself on your weight-loss success! You have achieved the weight you were aiming for and are likely to have permanently improved your health and retrained your eating habits.

▶ Because you now weigh less, your body needs fewer calories to function. The tried-and-tested 1-Day Maintenance Diet is designed to ensure that you keep the weight off.

▶ The 1-Day Maintenance Diet involves doing one restricted day every week, six days of an unrestricted Mediterranean diet, and maintaining your activity levels (300 minutes per week). This should enable you to keep your new weight stable.

▶ Key elements of successful maintenance are regular monitoring of your weight and serving sizes, staying active, setting a new goal and reward system for yourself, and getting the support you need.

▶ If your weight has plateaued and you would like to lose more, go back to the basics of The 2-Day Diet (see page 44) and repeat your goal setting and monitoring.

8

meal planners

Here are some suggested meal plans to help guide you through the early weeks of The 2-Day Diet—until the two-day pattern of eating becomes established. We've given you four weeks of menu suggestions with the restricted days falling on a Monday and Tuesday, as many of our Dieters chose these two days as their diet days. You can, of course, swap them around if other days work better for you. It is probably a good idea to try as much as possible to stick to the same two days each week so The 2-Day Diet becomes a habit. However, the beauty of the Diet is that you can move the days to fit into your week.

This chapter includes both standard and vegetarian plans that combine easy-to-prepare recipes with quick, healthy meals. When you reach the end of Week 4, you can go back to the beginning, adding in some of the other recipes that you'll find in chapters 9 and 10.

Use the planner in the way that works best for you. Some Dieters find that sticking closely to suggested meal plans helps them to keep focused, especially at the beginning of The 2-Day Diet. For those who want more flexibility, the meal plans will provide a great starting point to mix and match meal ideas. Drinks have not been included on these meal plans, but it is important to drink 2 quarts of low-calorie drinks (see page 56) per day. Two dairy portions have been included on each day, and it is assumed that one additional dairy portion will be used as milk in drinks throughout the day.

Week 1

Meal	Monday	Tuesday	Wednesday	Thursday	Friday	Saturday	Sunday
Breakfast	Grilled bacon and plum tomatoes Milky coffee	Recipe: Eggs on a bed of spinach	Recipe: Oatmeal with dried fruit	Shredded wheat cereal with milk	Bran-based cereal and milk	Whole grain toast, olive oil spread and low-sugar jam	Recipe: Classic muesli
Midmorning snack							Handful of Brazil nuts
Lunch	Recipe: Cauliflower soup	Vegetable crudités with low-fat hummus and low-fat cream cheese	Recipe: Tuna and white bean salad Yogurt	Recipe: Warm beet and feta salad, served with new potatoes	Recipe: Lentil soup with spinach and a touch of lemon, served with a chicken salad sandwich on whole wheat bread with low-fat mayonnaise	Whole wheat crackers with low-fat cream cheese plus a mixed salad with salmon and butter beans, with olive oil dressing	Rye toast with low-fat spread and baked beans
Midafternoon snack	Slice of melon	Handful of pistachio nuts	Apple	Handful of mixed unsalted nuts		Apple	Glass of vegetable juice
Evening meal	Recipe: Baked stuffed mackerel served with large serving of steamed broccoli	Recipe: Chicken or turkey stir-fry with snow peas and green beans Strawberries and yogurt	Recipe: Baked chicken with rosemary, served with bulgur wheat and three servings of steamed vegetables	Recipe: Beef meatballs with sauce and whole wheat spaghetti, served with a large mixed salad Recipe: Prune delight	Grilled trout served with new potatoes and two servings of steamed vegetables Recipe: Baked nectarines stuffed with nuts	Recipe: Chicken fajitas, served with a large mixed salad Recipe: Yogurt ice cream with raspberries	Recipe: Eggplant curry with chickpeas, rice, and a mango raita
Evening snack	Handful of almonds		Olives		Vegetable crudités and tomato salsa		Clementine, small glass of low-fat milk

Week 2

Meal	Monday	Tuesday	Wednesday	Thursday	Friday	Saturday	Sunday
Breakfast	Half a grapefruit; Recipe: Spicy scrambled eggs	Recipe: Papaya and golden flaxseed smoothie	Bran flakes and milk	Whole grain toast with peanut butter	Shredded wheat with milk	Smoked salmon with whole wheat toast and spread	Recipe: Oatmeal with dried fruit
Midmorning snack			Grapes		Fat-free yogurt		Pear
Lunch	Recipe: Zingy smoked salmon salad with avocado	Recipe: Chinese vegetable soup with tofu	Recipe: Creamy mushroom soup, served with a ham and lettuce sandwich on whole wheat roll with low-fat spread; Yogurt	Recipe: White bean salad with hard-boiled eggs, served with whole wheat crackers and low-fat cream cheese	Whole grain toast with low-fat spread and a can of sardines in tomato sauce; Glass of vegetable juice	Recipe: Horiatiki salata—Greek salad, served with whole wheat bread	Recipe: Zucchini soup with basil and tomato salsa, and a chicken and lettuce sandwich on a whole wheat roll
Midafternoon snack	Piece of Edam	Handful of Brazil nuts	Two clementines		Small apple	Handful of mixed unsalted nuts	
Evening meal	Recipe: Tangy chicken drumsticks with crudités and a harissa dip	Recipe: White fish with tangy watercress sauce, served with two servings of steamed vegetables	Recipe: Shrimp with beans, tomatoes, and thyme, served with brown rice and a mixed green salad	Olives; Recipe: Marinated lamb and red onion kebabs with a yogurt and herb sauce, served with new potatoes and a large mixed salad or three servings of vegetables; Recipe: Apricot and apple fruit salad	Recipe: Zucchini frittata, served with baked potato and mixed salad beans; Frozen yogurt with raspberries	Recipe: Chicken tagine with carrots and chickpeas, served with couscous; Fruit and yogurt	Recipe: Roasted vegetables with broiled halloumi, served with homemade potato wedges and a green salad
Evening snack	Handful of pistachio nuts	Cherry tomatoes	Handful of unsalted peanuts				Yogurt

Week 3

Meal	Monday	Tuesday	Wednesday	Thursday	Friday	Saturday	Sunday
Breakfast	Recipe: Eggs on a bed of spinach	Grilled bacon and tomatoes with mushrooms fried in olive oil Milky coffee	Bran flakes with mixed seeds and milk	Scrambled egg and canned plum tomatoes on rye toast Glass of milk	Fruit and fiber cereal with milk	Whole grain toast and olive spread with mushrooms fried in olive oil, grilled tomatoes, and a poached egg	Bran-based cereal with chopped mixed nuts and milk
Midmorning snack				Pear		Plums	
Lunch	Recipe: Chicken soup Handful of unsalted mixed nuts	Tuna salad made with canned tuna and an olive oil dressing	Recipe: Roasted red pepper soup, served with whole grain bread and low-fat hummus Tangerines	Salmon and cucumber sandwiches made with canned salmon and whole wheat bread Yogurt	Recipe: Tabbouleh with low-fat hummus	Baked potato, baked beans, and grated low-fat cheddar	Recipe: A pair of potato salads (the smoked fish version) Strawberries and yogurt
Midafternoon snack	Summer berry smoothie made with frozen mixed berries, milk, yogurt, and vanilla		Yogurt		Apple, handful of pistachio nuts	Glass of vegetable juice	Recipe: Guacamole, served with carrot sticks
Evening meal	Recipe: Lamb chops and "little dishes"	Recipe: Quick cauliflower and okra curry with a yogurt and mint raita Strawberries	Recipe: Mediterranean chicken casserole, served with three servings of steamed vegetables and bulgur wheat Recipe: Chocolate and orange mousse	Recipe: Red pepper, zucchini, and mushroom lasagne, served with a side salad	Recipe: Bean and green pepper chili with brown rice Recipe: Crunchy blackberry and apple crumble, served with fat-free Greek yogurt	Corn on the cob, Recipe: Black pepper salmon, served with two servings of steamed vegetables Recipe: Crunchy blackberry and apple crumble	Recipe: Thai-style stir-fried beef with lime, red onion, and cucumber, served with whole wheat boiled noodles
Evening snack	Piece of smoked Gouda	Handful of unsalted Brazil nuts		Grapes			Dried apricots

Week 4

Meal	Monday	Tuesday	Wednesday	Thursday	Friday	Saturday	Sunday
Breakfast	Smoked white fish with grilled tomatoes	Recipe: Greek yogurt with blackberries and cinnamon-toasted cashews	Recipe: Oatmeal with dried fruit	Shredded wheat with milk	Bran flakes and milk Glass of pineapple juice	Whole wheat toast and peanut butter	Recipe: Classic muesli
Midmorning snack				Pear		Glass of milk	Apricot
Lunch	Recipe: Iced cucumber soup Piece of low-fat cheddar and piece of smoked Gouda	Ham and low-fat cottage cheese salad Handful of walnuts	Grilled chicken breast salad (lettuce, cucumber, and tomatoes) served with rye crisps and low-fat cream cheese	Recipe: Creamy mushroom soup, served with rye crisps and low-fat hummus Banana	Recipe: Zucchini soup with basil and a tomato salsa Sliced egg salad sandwich on whole grain bread	Baked potato with tuna and low-fat mayonnaise, served with a green salad	Baked beans with whole grain toast with grated low-fat cheddar
Midafternoon snack	Handful of pistachio nuts	Boiled egg and cherry tomatoes	Glass of vegetable juice			Recipe: tzatziki, served with cucumber and red pepper crudités	Glass of vegetable juice
Evening meal	Recipe: Pan-grilled turkey cutlets with garlic spinach Slice of melon	Recipe: Shrimp and vegetable kebabs	Recipe: Salmon with lentils, served with two servings of steamed vegetables or a large mixed salad Recipe: Crêpe, with honey	Chili made with ground sirloin and red kidney beans, served with brown rice, a dollop of plain yogurt, and a tomato and cucumber salad	Recipe: Baked chicken with rosemary, served with boiled potatoes in their skins and two servings of steamed vegetables Fruit and fat-free Greek yogurt	Recipe: Eggplant curry with chickpeas, rice (or a whole wheat chapati), and a mango raita Recipe: Baked nectarines stuffed with nuts	Recipe: Smoked fish cakes, served with a mixed salad
Evening snack			2 clementines	Handful of unsalted peanuts		Banana	

Week 1 (vegetarian)

Meal	Monday	Tuesday	Wednesday	Thursday	Friday	Saturday	Sunday
Breakfast	Poached eggs and plum tomatoes	Recipe: Eggs on a bed of spinach	Shredded wheat cereal with milk and dried fruit	Recipe: Oatmeal with dried fruit	Whole wheat toast and olive spread with grilled vegetarian sausages, grilled tomatoes, and mushrooms fried in olive oil Glass of orange juice	Recipe: Classic muesli	Whole wheat toast, olive spread, and low-sugar jam
Midmorning snack	Tofu strips sautéed in spices		Handful of pistachios				
Lunch	Recipe: Cauliflower soup	Vegetable crudités with low-fat hummus and low-fat cream cheese	Recipe: Zucchini soup with basil, served with rye crisps and hummus	Rye crisps with low-fat cream cheese plus a mixed salad with mixed beans and olive oil dressing	Recipe: Lentil soup with spinach and a touch of lemon, served with rye crisps or a slice of whole wheat bread and olive spread	Rye toast with low-fat spread and baked beans or Recipe: Boston baked beans	Boiled egg and butter bean salad (lettuce, spring onions, and tomatoes) with olive oil dressing
Midafternoon snack	Glass of milk	Handful of mixed unsalted nuts	Apple	Glass of vegetable juice	Yogurt	Low-fat hummus with celery and cucumber crudités	
Evening meal	Recipe: Oriental vegetable stir-fry with marinated tofu and cashews Stewed rhubarb with sweeteners added to taste, with fat-free Greek yogurt	Recipe: Italian bean stew Strawberries and yogurt	Recipe: Pasta arrabbiata with tofu, served with two servings of steamed vegetables Yogurt	Recipe: Homemade classic burgers (V alternative), with new potatoes and two servings of steamed vegetables Recipe: Yogurt ice cream with raspberries	Homemade pizza—use a whole wheat pizza base and a tomato purée, olive oil, and garlic base with vegetables (onions, peppers, corn, mushrooms, olives) and mozzarella cheese on top. Serve with a large salad.	Recipe: Warm beet and feta salad; served with new potatoes and sliced egg Clementine	Recipe: Eggplant curry with chickpeas, rice, and a mango raita Recipe: Prune delight, served with yogurt
Evening snack	Handful of unsalted peanuts	Boiled eggs	Olives		Peach	Handful of Brazil nuts	

Week 2 (vegetarian)

Meal	Monday	Tuesday	Wednesday	Thursday	Friday	Saturday	Sunday
Breakfast	Half a grapefruit Recipe: Spicy scrambled eggs	Recipe: Papaya and golden flaxseed smoothie	Bran flakes and milk	Whole grain toast with peanut butter	Shredded wheat cereal with milk Glass of fruit juice	Whole wheat toast and poached egg	Recipe: Oatmeal with dried fruit and honey
Midmorning snack	Piece of Edam	Boiled egg			Fat-free yogurt		Plum
Lunch	Recipe: Mint, feta, and soy-bean salad	Recipe: Chinese vegetable soup with tofu	Recipe: Creamy mushroom soup, served with whole wheat crackers and low-fat hummus Handful of unsalted peanuts	Recipe: White bean salad with hard-boiled eggs, served with whole grain crackers and low-fat soft white cheese	Recipe: Zucchini soup with basil and a tomato salsa, served with whole grain crackers and low-fat hummus	Recipe: Horiatiki salata (Greek salad), served with whole grain bread	Recipe: Boston baked beans, served with baked potato
Midafternoon snack	Handful of Brazil nuts		Pear	Cherry tomatoes	Banana		Low-fat cream cheese with carrot and cucumber sticks
Evening meal	Recipe: Ginger, soy, and chili tofu skewers with Chinese cabbage and snow pea salad	Recipe: Cauliflower and mushroom curry with yogurt (add tofu if you want extra bulk)	Recipe: Bean and green pepper chili, served with a green salad Fruit and yogurt	Olives Recipe: Crunchy stuffed peppers with arugula and raita, served with (recipe) Red cabbage coleslaw with nuts and seeds Recipe: Apricot and apple fruit salad	Bean and vegetable bake (Adapted recipe: Shrimp with beans, tomatoes, and thyme—make this without shrimp and instead soften onions and peppers in the oil before adding the tomatoes, and serve with a mashed potato topping)	Recipe: Zucchini frittata, served with baked potato and salad with mixed salad beans Recipe: Crunchy blackberry and apple crumble, served with yogurt	Recipe: Orzotto with peas and broad beans
Evening snack		Handful of mixed unsalted nuts		Glass of milk			Handful of walnuts

Week 3 (vegetarian)

Meal	Monday	Tuesday	Wednesday	Thursday	Friday	Saturday	Sunday
Breakfast	Recipe: Greek yogurt with blackberries and cinnamon-toasted cashews	Recipe: Eggs on a bed of spinach	Fruit and fiber cereal and milk	Scrambled egg and canned plum tomatoes on rye toast Glass of milk	Whole grain toast with olive spread, with mushrooms fried in olive oil, grilled tomatoes, and a poached egg	Bran flakes with mixed seeds and milk	Muesli and milk
Midmorning snack						Banana smoothie made with 1% milk and plain yogurt	
Lunch	Recipe: Cauliflower soup Tofu strips stir-fried in spices with sesame seeds	Mozzarella and tomato salad served with a green salad and olive oil dressing	Vegetarian sausage sandwich on a whole wheat roll, with a large side salad	Recipe: A pair of potato salads (the vegetarian version) Mixed pepper sticks and lowfat hummus	Recipe: Roast red pepper soup, served with rye crisps and low-fat hummus	Recipe: White bean salad with hard-boiled eggs, served with a slice of whole wheat bread and low-fat spread	Low-fat hummus and grated carrot sandwiches on whole grain bread, with a side salad Strawberries and yogurt
Midafternoon snack	Handful of almonds	Glass of vegetable juice		Kiwi fruit		Apple	Handful of unsalted mixed nuts
Evening meal	Recipe: Fluffy omelette with scallions and cheese served with a large mixed salad	Recipe: Oriental vegetable stir-fry with marinated tofu and cashews Slice of melon	Recipe: Bean and green pepper chili with brown basmati rice or a whole wheat chapati and low-fat plain yogurt to serve Recipe: Apricot and apple fruit salad	Recipe: Pasta arrabbiata with tofu, served with a side salad Banana and yogurt	Corn on the cob Recipe: Roasted vegetables with grilled halloumi Recipe: Crunchy blackberry and apple crumble and 1 portion of custard (sweeten to taste with sweeteners)	Recipe: Red pepper, zucchini, and mushroom lasagne, served with a large salad	Recipe: Baked eggs Tunisian style Recipe: Chocolate and orange mousse
Evening snack	Low-fat cottage cheese and crudités	Low-fat hummus and crudités					Plum

Week 4 (vegetarian)

Meal	Monday	Tuesday	Wednesday	Thursday	Friday	Saturday	Sunday
Breakfast	Grilled vegetarian sausages and tomatoes	Recipe: Spicy scrambled eggs	Recipe: Oatmeal with dried fruit	Shredded wheat cereal with milk	Grilled vegetarian sausage sandwich on a whole wheat roll with grilled tomatoes; Glass of milk	Fruit and fiber cereal and milk; Glass of pineapple juice	Tomato omelette with whole wheat toast and low-fat spread
Midmorning snack	Boiled egg	Apricots		Orange		Recipe: Guacamole, served with crudités	
Lunch	Recipe: Iced cucumber soup; Spiced stir-fried tofu strips	Recipe: Mint, feta, and soy-bean salad	Baked beans on whole grain toast	Sliced egg and lettuce whole wheat sandwich on granary bread, served with (recipe) Red cabbage coleslaw with nuts and seeds	Rye crisps served with olives, low-fat hummus, and vegetable crudités	Poached egg and granary toast soldiers	Recipe: Creamy mushroom soup, served with rye crisps with low-fat cream cheese and cucumber
Midafternoon snack	Handful of pistachio nuts	Handful of Brazil nuts	Cherry tomatoes	Banana		Slice of melon	Pear
Evening meal	Recipe: Stuffed portobello mushrooms; Slice of melon	Recipe: Ginger, soy, and chili tofu skewers with Chinese cabbage and snow pea salad	Recipe: Crunchy stuffed peppers with arugula and raita, served with tomato salsa; Fruit and yogurt	Recipe: Zucchini frittata, served with steamed vegetables; Recipe: Lemon and honey cheesecake	Recipe: Bean and green pepper chili, served with brown rice; Recipe: Baked nectarines stuffed with nuts, served with yogurt	Recipe: Roasted vegetables with broiled halloumi, served with quinoa; Recipe: Crêpe with honey	Adapted recipe: Italian bean stew with TVP added to the tomatoes and a mashed potato topping served with steamed vegetables; Recipe: Lemon and blueberry yogurt cake
Evening snack		Low-fat cottage cheese and cucumber sticks		Glass of vegetable juice			

9

recipes for the two restricted days

General note

Most of these recipes serve one or two people. If you are increasing quantities to feed more people, bear in mind that you may also need to adjust the cooking time. In some cases, making a single portion is impractical—curries, soups, and stews, especially—and any excess can always be frozen so you have a stock of healthy frozen meals.

All spoon measurements are level unless otherwise indicated and are assumed to be standard sizes: 1 teaspoon = 5 ml; 1 tablespoon = 15 ml. If you have any doubt, get a set of measuring spoons.

All stove tops and ovens differ, so do check as you cook. The oven temperatures given are for conventional electric ovens and gas ovens; for convection ovens, subtract 25°F from the suggested cooking temperature.

Salt and sugar

Many of us have developed a preference for salty and sugary foods because of years of eating salty and sweet manufactured foods or habitually adding salt and sugar to flavor our food. Reducing salt and sugar intake is an important component of healthy eating. Cutting down on salt and sugar is quite straightforward: you simply need to get used to eating less.

Initially, when you reduce your salt and sugar intake, foods may taste bland or different. You can cut down on salt right away or reduce your salt intake in 20 percent steps. Most people can't taste the difference if they reduce salt gradually. Either way, after two or three weeks you will start to taste the genuine, delicious flavors of food. The recipes below include lots of alternative flavorings and do not require salt.

Some recipes contain stock, and we suggest that you use no more than 2 g or ¼ stock cube per serving. You can use less than this if you wish or a low-salt bouillon. Try to use tuna and beans canned in water, not brine or salted water. Similarly, try to use raw shrimp, rather than cooked, as these contain much less salt: 3½ oz (100 g) of cooked shrimp typically contain 1.1–2 g salt, whereas raw shrimp contain 0.5 g.

Recipes for your two restricted days

Breakfast	Page
Greek yogurt with blackberries and cinnamon-toasted cashews (V)	183
Spicy scrambled eggs (V)	183
Smoked salmon and spinach wraps with cottage cheese and lemon	184
Eggs on a bed of spinach (V)	185
Papaya and golden flaxseed smoothie (V)	186
Soups	
Hot and sour shrimp soup	186
Chinese vegetable soup with tofu (V)	187

Each recipe shows how many servings it contributes to your allowance in The 2-Day Diet plan. Many foods contain a combination of nutrients, some of which are in such small quantities they do not count toward your serving allowances. All servings have been rounded to the nearest half.

Breakfast

Greek yogurt with blackberries and cinnamon-toasted cashews

Serves 1

10 unsalted cashew nuts
pinch of ground cinnamon
4 oz (120 g) low-fat Greek
*   yogurt*
2 oz (80 g) blackberries

SERVINGS		NUTRITIONAL INFO	
Protein	0	Calories	172
Fat	1	Carbohydrate	15 g
Dairy	1	Protein	9 g
Fruit	1	Fiber	5 g
Vegetables	0	Salt	0.3 g

Place a small frying pan over medium heat. When hot, add the cashews and cinnamon to the pan and toast for 1–2 minutes, stirring occasionally with a wooden spoon, until golden and aromatic. Remove onto a chopping board and when cool enough to handle, roughly chop the nuts.

Spoon the yogurt into a bowl and top with the blackberries. Finish by sprinkling with the cinnamon cashews.

Spicy scrambled eggs

Serves 1

2 eggs
½ tsp canola oil
3 scallions, chopped
½ mild chili or to taste, finely
*   chopped (optional)*
¼ tsp turmeric
handful of cilantro leaves
1 medium tomato, chopped

SERVINGS		NUTRITIONAL INFO	
Protein	2	Calories	228
Fat	0	Carbohydrate	4 g
Dairy	0	Protein	17 g
Fruit	0	Fiber	2 g
Vegetables	1½	Salt	0.5 g

Beat the eggs in a mug or bowl with a tablespoon of water.

Put the oil in a small nonstick pan over medium heat. When hot, add the scallions and chili (if using) to the pan, and cook gently until the scallions just begin to color.

Add the turmeric and cilantro to the pan and stir for a few seconds, then add the tomato and continue stirring until the tomato is warmed through. Finally, add the beaten eggs and cook, stirring constantly, until the eggs begin to set. Remove the pan from the heat and serve immediately.

Smoked salmon and spinach wraps with cottage cheese and lemon

Serves 1

2 oz (60 g) smoked salmon slices
1 cup (2½ oz) baby spinach, washed and thoroughly dried
⅓ cup (75 g) low-fat cottage cheese
zest of half a lemon
black pepper

SERVINGS		NUTRITIONAL INFO	
Protein	2	Calories	181
Fat	0	Carbohydrate	4 g
Dairy	1	Protein	27 g
Fruit	0	Fiber	2 g
Vegetables	1	Salt	3.7 g

Lay the slices of smoked salmon out onto a chopping board and sprinkle with the spinach leaves, making sure to contain them within the edges of the salmon slices. Spoon some cottage cheese along the center of each slice and season with the lemon zest and a grind of black pepper. Roll up each salmon slice and serve immediately.

Eggs on a bed of spinach

Serves 1

1½ cups (3½ oz) baby
spinach leaves
black pepper
dash of vinegar
2 eggs

SERVINGS		NUTRITIONAL INFO	
Protein	2	Calories	210
Fat	0	Carbohydrate	2 g
Dairy	0	Protein	18 g
Fruit	0	Fiber	3 g
Vegetables	1	Salt	0.8 g

Wash the spinach leaves and chop them roughly. Put the leaves into a pan over a medium heat, add a couple of grinds of black pepper, cover, and cook until the spinach begins to wilt. The water clinging to the leaves after washing will provide enough moisture to cook the spinach. Only cook the leaves until they have wilted down.

Fill a small pan with about ½ in of water and add a little vinegar. Bring the water to the boil. Crack each egg into a cup. When the water is boiling, slide the eggs into the pan and reduce the heat to a simmer (if you are using an electric stove, you can switch the burner off). Cover the pan and allow the eggs to poach until they are done to your taste—3 minutes or so should produce a set white and a runny yolk.

Drain the spinach well, put it on a warmed plate, and spread it out. Lift the eggs from the pan with a slotted spoon so the water drains away and place them on top of the spinach. Add a little pepper to taste and serve immediately.

Papaya and golden flaxseed smoothie
Serves 1

½ cup (120 g) low-fat plain
    yogurt
juice of half a lime
⅓ cup (80 g) ripe papaya,
    skinned and deseeded
5 ice cubes
1 tsp golden flaxseeds

SERVINGS		NUTRITIONAL INFO	
Protein	0	Calories	112
Fat	½	Carbohydrate	14 g
Dairy	1	Protein	7 g
Fruit	1	Fiber	3 g
Vegetables	0	Salt	0.2 g

Pour the yogurt and lime juice into a blender and add the papaya. Blend until smooth (alternatively, use a stick blender) and pour into a large glass over ice. Sprinkle with the flaxseeds and serve immediately.

Soups

Hot and sour shrimp soup
Serves 1

1½ cups (12 fl oz) low-salt
    fish or vegetable stock
½ tsp fish sauce (optional)
1 small red chili, finely chopped
juice of half a lime
½ tsp low-salt soy sauce
½-in piece of fresh ginger
    root, finely grated
1 stick lemongrass, outer leaves
    removed, finely sliced
6 oz (180 g) raw jumbo shrimp

SERVINGS		NUTRITIONAL INFO	
Protein	4	Calories	175
Fat	0	Carbohydrate	5 g
Dairy	0	Protein	35 g
Fruit	0	Fiber	2 g
Vegetables	1	Salt	2.1 g

1 scallion, finely sliced
3 cherry tomatoes, halved
7 button mushrooms, halved
1 tbsp chopped cilantro

Pour the hot fish stock into a saucepan and add the fish sauce, chili, lime juice, soy sauce, ginger, and lemongrass and place over medium heat. Bring to a boil, lower the heat, and simmer for 3–4 minutes, until fragrant. Add the shrimp, scallions, tomatoes, and mushrooms and simmer for 2 more minutes, until the shrimp have turned pink. Serve immediately, sprinkled with the cilantro.

Chinese vegetable soup with tofu

Serves 1

1 cup (8 fl oz) low-salt vegetable stock
1 small pak choi or half a large one, trimmed (about 2 oz/60 g)
3 button mushrooms, finely sliced
3 scallions, trimmed and finely sliced
1 small slice fresh ginger root (about ¼ inch thick)

1 garlic clove
5 oz (150 g) firm tofu
dash of light soy sauce

SERVINGS		NUTRITIONAL INFO	
Protein	3	Calories	149
Fat	0	Carbohydrate	6 g
Dairy	0	Protein	15 g
Fruit	0	Fiber	4 g
Vegetables	1½	Salt	1.2 g

Put the stock in a pan and bring it to the boil. Separate the pak choi leaves, then slice the stems into thin sticks and the leaves into strips. Put the stems into the stock, together with the mushrooms and the scallions and lower the heat to a simmer. Grate the ginger and garlic into the pan and cook for 3 minutes.

Cut the tofu into pieces about ½-in square. Add the sliced pak choi leaves to the pan and stir them in. Then gently put the tofu in the pan and simmer for another 2 minutes.

Take the pan off the heat, then, using a slotted spoon, lift the vegetables and tofu into a serving bowl. Carefully pour the liquid on top and serve immediately with a dash of light soy sauce.

Tip:

℘ Not suitable for freezing.

Cauliflower soup
Serves 1, generously

1 small cauliflower
(about 7 oz /200 g)
½ tsp canola oil
½ leek, chopped
1 garlic clove, crushed
2 cups (16 fl oz) low-salt
vegetable stock
about ½ cup (4 fl oz) 1% or
fat-free milk
black pepper

SERVINGS		NUTRITIONAL INFO	
1% milk			
Protein	0	Calories	182
Fat	0	Carbohydrate	17 g
Dairy	½	Protein	14 g
Fruit	0	Fiber	7 g
Vegetables	3½	Salt	1.1 g

Trim the outer leaves from the cauliflower and split it into florets, cutting away the central stalk—there should be 6 oz/ 175 g of cauliflower remaining.

Heat the oil in a pan and add the leek. Stir it for a minute, then add the cauliflower florets and the garlic. Stir these around for 1 more minute, but don't let them brown; then add the stock. Bring the stock to the boil, reduce the heat, and simmer uncovered, until the cauliflower and leek are soft and the liquid is much reduced—about 15 minutes.

Remove the pan from the heat. Blend the soup using a handheld blender or place the contents in a blender and blitz, adding enough milk to reach a consistency you like. Return the soup to the pan (if you've used a blender), add black pepper to taste, then reheat and serve.

Tip:

∞ This simple and delicious soup is suitable for making in batches and freezing—just multiply the ingredients as required.

Chicken soup
Serves 1

1 chicken breast, skin removed, about 5 oz (150 g)
2 cups (16 fl oz) low-salt vegetable stock
1 small bay leaf
sprig of thyme
1 leek, trimmed
3 green or broad beans, cut into ½-in lengths

SERVINGS		NUTRITIONAL INFO	
Protein	5	Calories	239
Fat	0	Carbohydrate	9 g
Dairy	0	Protein	39 g
Fruit	0	Fiber	6 g
Vegetables	3	Salt	1.2 g

about ¼ cup (2 fl oz)
1% milk (optional)
black pepper

Put the whole chicken breast into a pan with the stock. Add the bay leaf and thyme sprig, bring the stock to a boil, then reduce the heat and simmer for 10 minutes.

Divide the leek into green and white parts, then chop the green part and add it to the pan. Simmer for 10 more minutes. While simmering, chop the rest of the leek and add to the stock with the beans.

Continue simmering for 5 more minutes, by which time the chicken should be tender and cooked through; cook a little longer if necessary.

Carefully lift the chicken out of the pan with a slotted spoon and chop it into cubes no larger than ½ in. Remove the bay leaf and the woody stem of the thyme sprig from the stock. Return the chicken pieces to the pan and increase the temperature to reduce the liquid and reheat the chicken. This will take about 5 minutes.

To serve you can either:

▶ Eat the soup as it is with small cubes of chicken and vegetables in a beautifully flavored broth.

▶ Ladle the liquid and some of the vegetables into a tall sturdy container, add the milk, blitz together with a handheld blender, then return the liquid to the pan.

▶ Add the milk to the pan and blend everything together into a smooth soup using a handheld blender (or blitz using a blender and return to the pan).

Whatever you decide, reheat the soup and season with black pepper before serving.

Tips:

▶ You could replace the beans with another green vegetable (see page 53).

▶ This soup is suitable for making in batches and freezing— simply multiply the ingredients as required.

Iced cucumber soup

Serves 1

½ *small cucumber, peeled and chopped*
½ *leek, trimmed and chopped*
½ *tsp canola oil*
½ *cup (4 fl oz) 1% milk*
½ *tsp cornstarch*
½ *cup (4 fl oz) low-salt vegetable stock*
a few fresh chives, chopped
black pepper

SERVINGS		NUTRITIONAL INFO	
Protein	0	Calories	138
Fat	0	Carbohydrate	17 g
Dairy	1	Protein	7 g
Fruit	0	Fiber	3 g
Vegetables	3	Salt	0.7 g

Prepare the cucumber and leek, then heat the oil in a pan over medium heat and add the chopped vegetables. Put the milk in a separate pan and warm it up.

Cover the pan with the cucumber and leeks and cook gently for about 5 minutes—check to make sure there is no sign of burning. Put the cornstarch in a small bowl and add a little of the hot milk. Blend together until you have a smooth paste and then add it to the pan of vegetables. Stir well for a minute or so and then take the pan off the heat.

Gradually stir in the rest of the hot milk and the stock. Return the pan to the heat and bring it to a boil, then reduce the heat and simmer gently for 20 minutes. Blend the soup thoroughly and transfer it to a bowl when it is completely smooth (it should have the consistency of cream). Allow the soup to cool, then cover the bowl and chill the soup in the refrigerator until completely cold.

When you are ready to serve, take the bowl out of the refrigerator and scatter some chopped chives over the surface. Add a little black pepper and serve immediately.

Tip:

    ⅚ This soup needs to be eaten fresh and is not suitable for freezing. The cornstarch provides 1 g of carbohydrate.

Japanese miso soup with shiitake mushrooms and greens
Serves 1

½ tbsp good-quality miso paste
1¼ cups (10 fl oz) freshly boiled water
½ tsp soy sauce
¼-in piece fresh ginger root, finely grated
2 scallions, finely sliced
¾ cup (1½ oz) green spinach, washed

3 asparagus spears, sliced into ½-in pieces
3 shiitake mushrooms, sliced
¼ tsp toasted sesame seeds

SERVINGS		NUTRITIONAL INFO	
Protein	0	Calories	59
Fat	0	Carbohydrate	5 g
Dairy	0	Protein	5 g
Fruit	0	Fiber	4 g
Vegetables	1½	Salt	1.2 g

Put the miso paste in a small bowl and add 2–3 tablespoons of the boiling water to make a paste. Spoon the paste into a small saucepan and gradually stir in the remaining water to make a smooth stock. Add the soy sauce and ginger and bring to a boil. Lower the heat and simmer for 2–3 minutes before adding the scallions, spinach, asparagus, and mushrooms. Simmer for 2 minutes, add the sesame seeds, and serve immediately.

Salads and light bites

Dips
Tzatziki
Serves 1

½ cup (4 oz) low-fat or
    fat-free Greek yogurt
1 small garlic clove, crushed
2-in piece of cucumber, peeled
large handful of cilantro
    leaves
half a handful of mint leaves
black pepper

SERVINGS		NUTRITIONAL INFO	
Protein	0	Calories	103
Fat	0	Carbohydrate	15 g
Dairy	1	Protein	10 g
Fruit	0	Fiber	1 g
Vegetables	1	Salt	0.3 g

Put the yogurt and crushed garlic into a bowl. Slice the cucumber in half and remove the seeds with a spoon, then finely chop the flesh. Add this to the yogurt mixture.

    Chop the cilantro and mint leaves together and add them to the yogurt, then stir everything together. Grind some black pepper on top and serve immediately.

Guacamole
Serves 1

½ ripe avocado	SERVINGS		NUTRITIONAL INFO	
squeeze of lemon juice	Protein	0	Calories	155
1 scallion, chopped	Fat	2	Carbohydrate	4 g
4 cherry tomatoes, chopped	Dairy	0	Protein	2 g
½ small red chili (or to	Fruit	0	Fiber	5 g
taste), finely chopped	Vegetables	½	Salt	< 0.1 g

Remove the pit from the avocado. Slice through the flesh just to the skin lengthwise, and then do the same across. Then bend the avocado back on itself—the flesh will either come out or will be very easy to remove, depending on its ripeness.

Put it in a bowl, add a little lemon juice, and mash the flesh with a fork until there are no large pieces. Stir in the scallion, tomatoes, and chili, check for seasoning, and serve immediately.

Tip:
▶ Both these dips are great served with vegetable crudités or with iceberg lettuce leaves used as scoops.

Crab salad
Serves 1

6 oz (1 x 170 g) can of white	SERVINGS		NUTRITIONAL INFO	
crabmeat or 3½ oz	Protein	4	Calories	316
(100 g) fresh crabmeat	Fat	2½	Carbohydrate	4 g
2 tsp low-fat mayonnaise	Dairy	0	Protein	22 g
zest and juice of ½ lemon	Fruit	0	Fiber	5 g
few drops of Tabasco sauce	Vegetables	1	Salt	1.4 g
(optional)				

black pepper
3 scallions, trimmed and
   chopped

½ avocado, pit removed
handful of salad leaves
   (about 2 oz/60 g)

Drain the can of crab into a sieve, rinse under running water, and set the sieve over a bowl to drain thoroughly. Omit this step if you are using fresh crab, but check the crabmeat for any small pieces of shell.

Break up any chunks of crabmeat very gently, using a fork, and set aside.

Put the mayonnaise into a bowl and squeeze in a scant teaspoon of the lemon juice, then add the lemon zest to the mixture. Add the Tabasco, if using, and plenty of black pepper. Add the scallions and stir everything together.

Slice lengthwise through the flesh of the avocado just to the skin, and do the same across; then bend the avocado back on itself and remove the cubes of flesh. Put these in the bowl of mayonnaise and add the crabmeat. Turn all the ingredients together gently, but make sure everything is incorporated.

Put some salad leaves on a plate and spoon the crab salad on top. Serve immediately.

Tuna pâté with crudités
Serves 1

5½–6½ oz (1 x 160–185 g)
   can of solid white albacore
   tuna in spring water
1 heaping tbsp low-fat cream
   cheese
1 heaping tbsp low-fat or
   fat-free Greek yogurt

squeeze or two of lemon juice
drop or two of Tabasco or
   Worcestershire sauce, to
   taste
black pepper

For the crudités:

3 celery sticks, trimmed and
*　　cut into smaller sticks*
6 scallions, trimmed
2-in piece of cucumber,
*　　peeled, cut into strips*

SERVINGS		NUTRITIONAL INFO	
Protein	3½–4	Calories	228
Fat	0	Carbohydrate	7 g
Dairy	1½	Protein	35 g
Fruit	0	Fiber	4 g
Vegetables	3	Salt	0.6 g

Drain the can of tuna. If you could only buy fish in brine, put it in a sieve and rinse under running water to remove excess salt.

Transfer the tuna to a bowl and break it up with a fork, then add the cream cheese and the yogurt and mix together. Add a squeeze or two of lemon juice and, tasting carefully, a little Tabasco or Worcestershire sauce. Then add some black pepper and mix everything once more.

Cover the bowl and put the pâté in the refrigerator for at least 2 hours to allow the flavors to develop. Prepare the crudités just before serving.

Tips:

▶ This is a very adaptable recipe: for a firmer, more set pâté, use 2 cans of tuna; for a softer dip, use more yogurt. Either way, it is ideal for a packed lunch.

Zingy smoked salmon salad with avocado
Serves 1

2½ oz (75 g) smoked salmon
black pepper
1 lemon
½-in piece of cucumber,
*　　peeled*

1 tsp olive oil
½ tsp sesame seeds
small bunch watercress
small bunch arugula leaves
½ small avocado

Cut the smoked salmon into strips and put them in a bowl. Grind some black pepper over them and squeeze a little lemon juice over them as well; stir together. Cut the cucumber in half lengthwise and

SERVINGS		NUTRITIONAL INFO	
Protein	2	Calories	226
Fat	2½	Carbohydrate	2 g
Dairy	0	Protein	22 g
Fruit	0	Fiber	3 g
Vegetables	1	Salt	3.6 g

remove the seeds, then cut each half in half again lengthwise, and finely slice the cucumber sections. Add them to the smoked salmon. Set the bowl aside while you prepare the dressing and assemble the salad.

Put the olive oil in a small bowl and add a squeeze of lemon juice. Whisk or stir them together well and then scatter in the sesame seeds. Tear the leaves from the watercress stalks and put them on a serving plate with the arugula. Peel the avocado and cut it into fine slices. Put these around the salad, then spoon the salmon and cucumber mixture on top. Whisk up the dressing once more and drizzle it over the salad. Serve immediately.

Tip:

▶ As an alternative, make this salad using fresh horseradish instead of the sesame seeds—when it is in season. Grate a little fresh root into the dressing about 30 minutes before assembling the salad. Fresh horseradish can be found at farmers' markets, in good supermarkets, or online—and it's best in autumn and winter.

Fish and seafood

Chili and pesto red snapper
Serves 1

2 red snapper fillets, about
4 oz (120 g) each
½ red chili, finely chopped
1 tsp pesto
juice and zest of ½ a lemon
a small handful of torn basil
leaves, to serve

SERVINGS		NUTRITIONAL INFO	
Protein	4	Calories	254
Fat	1	Carbohydrate	3 g
Dairy	0	Protein	36 g
Fruit	0	Fiber	3 g
Vegetables	1	Salt	0.9 g

For the kale:
1½ cups shredded curly kale leaves

Preheat broiler to high.

Make 2 diagonal slices on the skin of each fillet and place on a rimmed baking tray. Mix together the chili, pesto, and half of the lemon juice and zest to make a marinade. Pour over the fish—making sure that it is completely smothered on both sides. Set aside for 20 minutes.

Meanwhile, sprinkle the remaining lemon juice and zest over the kale and massage the kale between your fingers to soften the pieces, until they are slightly wilted. Set aside.

Broil the fish for 3 minutes on each side, until cooked through and the skin is crisp and slightly charred. Serve immediately on a bed of kale and scatter the basil leaves on top.

Salmon parcels with aromatic salad

Serves 2

4 lemon slices

1 small onion, sliced into
   rings (for flavor only)

1 fennel bulb

2 salmon fillets, about 4 oz
   (120 g) each

1 bay leaf

sprig of thyme

2 handfuls of salad leaves

6 scallions, finely sliced

4-in piece of cucumber,
   peeled, finely sliced

2 tsp olive oil (not
   extra-virgin)

squeeze of lemon juice

black pepper

SERVINGS		NUTRITIONAL INFO	
Protein	4	Calories	276
Fat	½	Carbohydrate	4 g
Dairy	0	Protein	27 g
Fruit	0	Fiber	4 g
Vegetables	2	Salt	0.2 g

Preheat the oven to 400°F.

Take a large piece of foil and put two lemon slices in the middle of it. Scatter the onion rings over the center of the foil as well. Cut a vertical slice off the fennel bulb and add that too. Put the two salmon fillets on top and tuck the bay leaf and thyme sprig between them. Top each fillet with the remaining slices of lemon and bring the edges of the foil up around the fish and over the top. Fold the edges together to make a loose but well-sealed parcel.

Put the parcel in an ovenproof dish or roasting pan and cook for 15 minutes in the preheated oven. Remove the dish from the oven and carefully open the foil—the salmon should be almost cooked. Fold back the edges of the foil, exposing the fish, and remove the top two slices of lemon. Then put the dish back in the oven for another 5 minutes, or until the fish is cooked and opaque all the way through.

Remove the bay leaf and thyme, and carefully lift the salmon off the lemon, onion, and fennel (discard these, along with the salmon skin).

Set the fish aside to cool slightly, and prepare the salad. Finely slice the rest of the fennel bulb and combine with the salad leaves, scallions, and cucumber. Drizzle the olive oil over the salad, squeeze in the lemon juice, grind in some black pepper, then toss all the salad ingredients together. Serve immediately with the salmon.

Tip:

▶ This salmon is very good cold, perhaps served with the "Almost a céleri rémoulade" (see page 236) as an accompaniment instead of the fennel salad.

▶ Or try it with some lemon mayonnaise—put 1 tablespoon of low-fat mayonnaise in a small dish, grate in a little lemon zest, and mix well.

▶ For unrestricted days, serve with boiled new potatoes.

Baked cod with spinach and asparagus served with quick-pickled radishes and cucumber
Serves 1

*1 skinless cod fillet, about
4–6 oz (120–180 g)
juice of half a lemon
black pepper
1-in piece of cucumber,
peeled, cut in half
vertically and finely sliced*

SERVINGS		NUTRITIONAL INFO	
Protein	2–3	Calories	206
Fat	0	Carbohydrate	5 g
Dairy	0	Protein	39 g
Fruit	0	Fiber	5 g
Vegetables	2½	Salt	0.4 g

¼-in piece of fresh ginger
root, very finely sliced
5 radishes, finely sliced
1½ tsp rice wine vinegar

¼ tsp toasted sesame seeds
½ cup baby spinach
5 spears of asparagus, sliced
into 2-in pieces

Preheat the oven to 350°F.

Place the cod in a small ovenproof dish and sprinkle with the lemon juice. Season with black pepper and bake in the oven for 8–10 minutes, until the fish flakes easily.

Place the sliced cucumber, ginger, and radish in a small bowl and sprinkle with the vinegar and sesame seeds. Set aside while the cod cooks.

Meanwhile, steam the vegetables for 1–2 minutes, until the spinach has wilted and the asparagus is tender.

Serve the cod on a bed of the steamed vegetables and top with the pickles.

White fish with tangy watercress sauce
Serves 2

2 cod, flounder, or pollock
fillets, about 5 oz (150 g)
each
2 tsp olive oil

For the sauce:
bunch of watercress (about
1½ cups leaves)
handful of flat-leaf parsley
handful of basil leaves

SERVINGS		NUTRITIONAL INFO	
Protein	2½	Calories	184
Fat	½	Carbohydrate	1 g
Dairy	0	Protein	30 g
Fruit	0	Fiber	2 g
Vegetables	1	Salt	0.3 g

1 tsp olive oil
large squeeze of lemon juice
1 tbsp water

Make the sauce first. Strip off the watercress leaves, discarding the thickest parts of the stalks and any yellow leaves. Put the leaves in a large container or blender. Add the parsley and basil leaves, the olive oil, and a squeeze of lemon juice. If using a hand blender, pulse the leaves together for a few seconds and then add a little water; if you are using a blender, add some water at the start. Blend until the leaves are thoroughly chopped and there are no large pieces remaining, then pour into a small bowl.

To cook the fish: pat the fillets dry with paper towels. Using a nonstick frying pan, heat the olive oil over medium to low heat. When the oil is hot, add the fish fillets, skin side down. Cook the fillets for 3–5 minutes, depending on how thick they are, then carefully turn over and cook for a little longer until done. The total cooking time should be 5–10 minutes; the fish is ready when it flakes easily, revealing opaque flesh. Serve immediately, accompanied by some of the sauce (if you have made the sauce in a blender, you may need to drain off some excess liquid first).

Tips:

▶ This dish can be made with any firm white fish, and the sauce also goes well with oily fish, such as salmon.

▶ On unrestricted days, you could serve this with new potatoes.

Shrimp and vegetable kebabs

Serves 1

*5 oz (150 g) raw jumbo
shrimp
7 cherry tomatoes
10 button mushrooms
½ zucchini, sliced into rings
green salad leaves*

SERVINGS		NUTRITIONAL INFO	
Protein	3	Calories	215
Fat	1	Carbohydrate	5 g
Dairy	0	Protein	31 g
Fruit	0	Fiber	3 g
Vegetables	3	Salt	0.8 g

*For the marinade:
small handful of cilantro
    leaves
½ –1 green chili pepper (to
    taste), deseeded*

*2 tsp olive oil
2 tsp lemon or lime juice
black pepper*

First make the marinade. Very finely chop the cilantro leaves and the green chili and transfer them to a bowl. Add the oil and lemon juice and a good grinding of black pepper. Rinse the shrimp, drain them well, and add them to the marinade. Stir everything together, cover the bowl, and put it to one side for 30 minutes. If using bamboo skewers, soak them in water.

Thread the skewers, shaking excess marinade off the shrimp as you lift them out of the bowl, and alternating them with the tomatoes, mushrooms, and slices of zucchini (discard what remains of the marinade). Preheat the broiler to a very high heat, then lower it slightly and put the skewers under the heat—suspend them over a baking dish or roasting pan—for 5–6 minutes, until they begin to brown and crisp nicely, turning them during this time. Serve the kebabs as soon as they are ready, with a green salad.

Black pepper salmon with olives and tomatoes
Serves 1

10 black olives, pitted and
    quartered
7 cherry tomatoes, halved
1 tsp olive oil
1 salmon fillet,
    skin removed, about
    4 oz (120 g)
black pepper
handful of basil leaves

SERVINGS		NUTRITIONAL INFO	
Protein	4	Calories	299
Fat	1½	Carbohydrate	6 g
Dairy	0	Protein	26 g
Fruit	0	Fiber	4 g
Vegetables	1	Salt	0.6 g

To serve:
small handful of arugula
    leaves
balsamic vinegar

Prepare the olives (if they have been in brine, rinse them well first) and put them in a bowl. Add the halved cherry tomatoes to the bowl as well, then add half a teaspoon of olive oil and stir them together.

Pat the salmon fillet dry with paper towels. Put the remaining oil on a plate and grind lots of black pepper over it, then rub all sides of the salmon fillet in the oil-and-pepper mix.

Empty the olive-and-tomato mixture into a small nonstick pan over a low heat—they should just warm through rather than simmer or boil. Keep an eye on the pan to make sure the mixture isn't starting to burn, and take it off the heat if there is any sign that this might be happening; cover the pan to keep the mixture warm.

Preheat a ridged grill pan or a small nonstick frying pan over a high heat. When the pan is really hot, put the salmon in the pan. Turn it over after 3 minutes and cook the other side for another 2 minutes, then turn it again and repeat until cooked (the flesh should be completely opaque) and the edges are crisping up. Just before it is ready, add some torn basil leaves to the tomato and olives so that they wilt a little in the warmth of the pan.

Put the salmon fillet on a serving plate and spoon the warm tomato, olive, and basil mixture beside it. Accompany with a handful of arugula leaves drizzled with a little balsamic vinegar.

Fresh tuna steak with a tomato salsa
Serves 1

1 tsp olive oil
1 fresh tuna steak, about
  150 g (5 oz)
black pepper

For a salsa:
1 medium tomato
3 scallions, white only, finely
  chopped
1 tsp extra-virgin olive oil
squeeze of lemon juice
black pepper

small handful of basil leaves

To serve:
Salad leaves or a portion of
  steamed vegetables

SERVINGS		NUTRITIONAL INFO	
Protein	5	Calories	288
Fat	1	Carbohydrate	5 g
Dairy	0	Protein	37 g
Fruit	0	Fiber	3 g
Vegetables	1½	Salt	0.2 g

Make the salsa first. Cut the tomato into quarters, then finely chop the flesh into small cubes and put in a small bowl. Add the chopped scallions to the chopped tomatoes, then the olive oil and lemon juice. Stir the salsa and add black pepper. Cover the bowl and set it to one side for 20 minutes. When ready to serve, tear the basil leaves and stir them into the salsa.

To cook the tuna, put the oil in a small nonstick frying pan over high heat. Sprinkle both sides of the tuna steak very lightly with a little black pepper, then put in the pan when the oil is really hot and almost smoking. Cook the tuna for no more than 2 minutes before turning it over and cooking the other side. How long this takes will depend on how thick the steak is; check by making a small cut in the middle of the steak with a sharp knife. Part the cut slightly and see how pink it is inside. Tuna is best eaten rare, like a beefsteak, and should be slightly pink; cook it to taste, but be careful not to overcook it or it will be tough and chewy. Put the tuna steak on a serving plate and spoon the salsa over it. Accompany with a bowl of salad leaves or a portion of steamed vegetables.

Tips:

▶ As an alternative, use halibut of the same weight if you would rather not use tuna. Be careful to test that it is cooked, and it may take a little more oil as well.

▶ Add some finely chopped red chili and a little crushed garlic to the salsa for an extra kick.

Garlic shrimp
Serves 1

1 tsp olive oil

1 garlic clove, crushed

6 oz (180 g) raw jumbo
   shrimp

juice of 1 lemon

½–1 tsp paprika (to taste)

SERVINGS		NUTRITIONAL INFO	
Protein	4	Calories	178
Fat	½	Carbohydrate	3 g
Dairy	0	Protein	32 g
Fruit	0	Fiber	1 g
Vegetables	1	Salt	0.8 g

To serve:
iceberg lettuce leaves

Put the oil in a nonstick frying pan over very high heat. Add the garlic and cook very briefly, stirring it around so it does not burn. Then immediately add the shrimp and stir them in; cook them for a minute. Pour the lemon juice into the pan and add the paprika. Cook, stirring all the time, until the lemon juice has been taken up completely and the shrimp are pink—this should take no longer than 2 minutes.

Serve immediately, spooning the shrimp over iceberg lettuce leaves and wrapping them up as you eat.

Tips:

▶ This delicious Mediterranean dish can be adapted for unrestricted days. Add more lemon juice and cook it at a slightly lower temperature so the shrimp are cooked but there is still plenty of lemony, spicy sauce. Serve over rice instead of using the lettuce leaves.

▶ If you're using cooked shrimp instead of raw ones, add the lemon juice and paprika immediately after putting the shrimp in the pan.

Broiled flounder with a zucchini nest

Serves 1

1 flounder fillet, about 6 oz
   (180 g)
drop of olive oil
1 tsp olive oil spread
1 small zucchini
1 tbsp low-fat or fat-free
   Greek yogurt
zest and juice of half a lemon   black pepper

SERVINGS		NUTRITIONAL INFO	
Protein	3	Calories	209
Fat	1	Carbohydrate	5 g
Dairy	½	Protein	30 g
Fruit	0	Fiber	1 g
Vegetables	2	Salt	0.6 g

Preheat the broiler. Put a piece of foil large enough to hold the flounder onto a broiler pan. Lightly brush the oil onto the foil. Carefully lift the fish onto the foil, skin side down, and dot it with the olive oil spread.

While the broiler is heating, wipe the zucchini and peel it into fine strips with a potato peeler, then set these to one side. Put the yogurt into a small bowl and add some lemon zest and a very little of the juice. Stir the yogurt and lemon together well. Put a pot of water on to boil.

While waiting for the water to boil, slide the flounder under the broiler, but not too close (ideally, about 4 in away), and cook the fish for about 5–6 minutes, until the flesh is opaque and the edges are beginning to crisp a little.

After the fish has been cooking for about 2 minutes, put the zucchini ribbons into the boiling water and turn off the heat immediately. Leave them in the boiling water for no more than a minute, then drain them well. Add the zucchini ribbons to the lemony yogurt bowl, then quickly twist the ribbons into a nest with a fork, rather like spaghetti. Spoon the nest onto a serving plate and then add the cooked flounder, lifting it very carefully from the foil with a spatula or similar flat utensil. Add a little black pepper and serve immediately.

Baked stuffed mackerel
Serves 2

2 fresh mackerel, gutted and heads removed, about 7 oz (200 g) each
black pepper
several sprigs of thyme

SERVINGS		NUTRITIONAL INFO	
Protein	7	Calories	270
Fat	0	Carbohydrate	1 g
Dairy	0	Protein	23 g
Fruit	0	Fiber	< 1 g
Vegetables	0	Salt	0.2 g

½ lemon, sliced   *½ red onion, sliced*

1 tbsp lemon juice   *(for flavor only)*

Preheat the oven to 400°F. Tear off a large piece of foil and find an ovenproof dish big enough to hold the fish easily.

Place the fish in the middle of the sheet of foil. Season them, both inside and out, with lots of black pepper. Push the thyme into the cavities of the fish, then stuff them further with the slices of lemon and red onion. Bring the foil up around the two fish and add the lemon juice. Then fold the foil over the fish, making a parcel, and seal it tightly.

Carefully lift the parcel into the ovenproof dish and put it in the hot oven. Bake the mackerel for 25 minutes, then unwrap the parcel carefully, as steam will escape. Remove most of the stuffing, lift the fish onto plates, and serve immediately. (If you like, you can quickly remove the skin from the fish and lift off the fillets first.) Serve with a green salad or steamed spinach.

Chicken and turkey

Roast chicken Provençal
Serves 1

1 skinless chicken breast, about 4 oz (120 g), chopped into bite-size pieces

¼ tsp olive oil

½ tsp balsamic vinegar

SERVINGS		NUTRITIONAL INFO	
Protein	4	Calories	197
Fat	0	Carbohydrate	8 g
Dairy	0	Protein	32 g
Fruit	0	Fiber	6 g
Vegetables	2½	Salt	0.4 g

2 garlic cloves, skins left on
   and crushed with the back
   of a knife
7 cherry tomatoes, sliced in
   half
1 leek, diced

1 tsp capers, drained
½ tsp dried oregano
black pepper
half lemon
1½ oz (40 g) watercress,
   tough stalks removed

Preheat the oven to 400°F.

Put all the ingredients (apart from the lemon, pepper, and watercress) in an ovenproof dish and toss to combine all of the flavors. Season with black pepper and roast in the oven for 20 minutes, until the chicken pieces are cooked through and the ingredients are golden. Squeeze the juice of the half lemon over all and serve immediately with the watercress.

Cream cheese, sun-dried tomato, and chive-stuffed chicken with grilled fennel and zucchini

Serves 1

1 tbsp low-fat cream cheese
1 small garlic clove, crushed
2 sun-dried tomatoes, finely
   chopped
1 tsp finely chopped chives
black pepper
1 skinless chicken breast
   (about 4 oz)
½ tsp olive oil
zest of half a lemon
half a zucchini, sliced into
   half moons

1½ oz (40 g) fennel, sliced
   into ⅛-in slices

SERVINGS		NUTRITIONAL INFO	
Protein	4	Calories	253
Fat	0	Carbohydrate	5 g
Dairy	1	Protein	33 g
Fruit	0	Fiber	2 g
Vegetables	3	Salt	0.8 g

Preheat the oven to 350°F.

Mix the cream cheese, garlic, sun-dried tomatoes, and chives together in a small bowl. Season with black pepper. Make a 2-in incision in the thickest part of the side of the chicken breast, about 1 in deep. Using a teaspoon, feed the stuffing into the chicken breast and seal the meat back together using a toothpick. Transfer to a small ovenproof dish and bake in the oven for 20–25 minutes, until the chicken is completely cooked through and the juices run clear when the meat is cut in the thickest part.

While the chicken is cooking, heat a grill pan over high heat. Mix together the olive oil and lemon zest and brush over the vegetable slices—season with black pepper.

Grill the vegetable slices for 1–2 minutes on each side, until nicely charred. Remove from the pan and serve with the chicken breast.

Larb gai—Thai chicken salad
Serves 1

1 small garlic clove, crushed
3½ oz (100 g) ground
   chicken or turkey
¼ cup (2 fl oz) low-salt
   chicken or vegetable stock
squeeze of lime juice
4 scallions, trimmed, two
   sliced and two finely
   chopped
1 red chili, deseeded and
   finely chopped (or to taste)

SERVINGS		NUTRITIONAL INFO	
Protein	3½	Calories	143
Fat	0	Carbohydrate	5 g
Dairy	0	Protein	26 g
Fruit	0	Fiber	3 g
Vegetables	1½	Salt	0.4 g

sprig of mint   *whole iceberg lettuce leaves,*
handful of cilantro leaves   *about 2¾ oz (80 g), to serve*

Mix the crushed garlic with the ground chicken. Heat the stock in a small pot over high heat until it is bubbling well. Then add the chicken mixture. Stir it in and continue stirring until the stock has evaporated and the chicken has cooked; this should only take about 3–4 minutes (be careful not to over-cook the chicken, or it will be tough).

Once cooked, put the chicken into a bowl, then add the lime juice, scallions, and chili. Stir well. Strip the leaves from the mint stalk and chop them with the cilantro leaves. Add the chopped leaves to the bowl and stir through, then check for seasoning.

Serve immediately, on iceberg lettuce leaves.

Pan-grilled turkey cutlets with garlic spinach
Serves 1

1 turkey cutlet, about 4 oz
   total weight
½ tsp Dijon mustard
½ lemon
½ tsp olive oil
black pepper

SERVINGS		NUTRITIONAL INFO	
Protein	4	Calories	211
Fat	0	Carbohydrate	5 g
Dairy	0	Protein	35 g
Fruit	0	Fiber	6 g
Vegetables	2½	Salt	1.2 g

For the spinach:
3 cups (7 oz) fresh baby
   spinach leaves
1 garlic clove, crushed
nutmeg, to taste (optional)

Prepare the spinach first. Wash and remove any long stems, then chop it very roughly. Put it in a pot with the crushed garlic.

Before cooking the turkey cutlet, first press it down with your hands, flattening it out more. Then spread half the mustard over one side, smoothing it in with a knife or your fingers; turn the cutlet over and spread the rest of the mustard on the other side. Cut a couple of slices off the lemon, set aside, and then juice the rest.

Preheat a ridged grill pan or large nonstick frying pan. If using a grill pan, brush the oil quickly over the surface of the ridges; if using a frying pan, swirl the oil around to spread it out.

Just before cooking the turkey, put the pot of spinach over medium heat and add a little grated nutmeg to it.

Just as the oil starts to smoke in your frying pan or grill pan, put on the turkey steak. Cook it on one side for about 3 minutes, then turn over and cook the other side for roughly the same time; sprinkle the lemon juice over the surface as you turn it. While you cook the steak, give the spinach a stir as well.

Check to see if the turkey steak is cooked through, then drain the spinach thoroughly, check it for seasoning, and put it on a serving plate. Lift the cutlet onto the plate, season with black pepper, and put the lemon slices on the side for squeezing over the meat. Serve immediately.

Tandoori-style chicken with a shredded salad
Serves 1

1 large chicken breast,   *2 tbsp plain yogurt*
*   skin removed*   *½ tsp garam masala*
*   (about 5 oz/150 g)*   *½ tsp turmeric*

½ tsp paprika

¼ tsp cayenne pepper

To serve:

handful of iceberg lettuce,
  about 2¾ oz (80 g), finely
  shredded
2 scallions, finely shredded
  into strips
2½-in piece of cucumber,
  peeled, deseeded, and
  finely shredded

lemon juice, to taste

black pepper

SERVINGS		NUTRITIONAL INFO	
Protein	5	Calories	240
Fat	0	Carbohydrate	8 g
Dairy	1	Protein	39 g
Fruit	0	Fiber	2 g
Vegetables	0	Salt	0.5 g

Take the chicken and pierce it in several places with a sharp knife. Put the yogurt in a glass or ceramic bowl and add the spices, stirring them well together.

Put the chicken in the bowl and smear the yogurt mixture over it, massaging the mixture into the pierced holes. Cover the bowl with plastic wrap and leave it in the refrigerator for 8–12 hours or overnight; if prepared to this stage in the morning, the chicken will be perfect to cook in the evening.

Preheat the oven to 400°F. Shake any excess yogurt marinade off the chicken and discard it. Then put the chicken in a deep baking dish (it should be deeper than the chicken breast). Cover the dish with foil, making sure it isn't touching the chicken, and bake for 20 minutes. Remove the foil and cook for another 15–20 minutes, turning the breast over during this time. Test to see if it is done (the juices should run clear when the chicken is pierced).

Mix together the finely shredded iceberg lettuce, fine shreds of scallions, and cucumber in a bowl and squeeze some lemon juice over them. Add a little black pepper and toss the salad once more. Serve immediately with the hot chicken.

Tips:

▶ The chicken doesn't have to be baked—you can always broil it instead. Remember to turn the chicken over as it cooks. How long it takes will depend on your broiler, as individual types vary.

▶ Served cold, this chicken makes a good addition to a packed lunch; just allow it to cool, then refrigerate until needed.

Garlic and thyme chicken livers with mushrooms and broccoli in a cream cheese sauce
Serves 1

4 oz (120 g) chicken livers

1 tbsp low-fat cream
* cheese*

2 tbsp hot chicken stock

¼ tsp olive oil

2 spears broccolini, cut into
* ½-in slices*

1 clove garlic, crushed

1 tsp thyme leaves,
* chopped*

7 small cremini mushrooms,
* sliced*

black pepper

SERVINGS		NUTRITIONAL INFO	
Protein	4	Calories	203
Fat	0	Carbohydrate	5 g
Dairy	1	Protein	31 g
Fruit	0	Fiber	4 g
Vegetables	1½	Salt	0.6 g

Begin by picking over the chicken livers, slicing off any bits of fat and sinew. Pat dry. Mix the cream cheese with the chicken stock and set aside. Heat the oil in a frying pan over medium heat. When the oil is hot, add the livers and the broccolini and fry for 2 minutes, until the livers have browned on all sides. Add the garlic, thyme, and mushrooms and continue to fry for another 2 minutes, until everything is nicely golden. Turn the heat down to low and pour in the cream-cheese-and-stock mixture. Allow to bubble for 30 seconds before removing from the heat. Serve seasoned with lots of black pepper.

Chicken cutlet with paprika and herbs
Serves 1

1 chicken breast, skin removed, about 5 oz (150 g)
1 tsp paprika
1 tsp dried mixed herbs
½ tsp olive oil

SERVINGS		NUTRITIONAL INFO	
Protein	5	Calories	199
Fat	0	Carbohydrate	3 g
Dairy	0	Protein	35 g
Fruit	0	Fiber	2 g
Vegetables	2	Salt	0.4 g

To serve:
bowlful of green salad, about 1 cup
handful of arugula leaves, about ⅓ cup
6 radishes, trimmed and halved
2 lemon slices
black pepper

Tear off a large piece of parchment paper and fold it in half, then open it up. Remove any excess fat from the chicken and put the chicken breast on one half of the paper; fold the other half on top of it. Take a rolling pin or similar heavy item and whack the chicken breast, flattening it until it is no thicker than ¼ in. Put the paprika and herbs on a plate and mix them together thoroughly.

Heat the oil in a small nonstick frying pan over medium heat. When it is hot, take the chicken breast and dip one side into the spice-and-herb mix, then flip it over and do the other side. Put the chicken cutlet into the frying pan and cook it for 3–4 minutes—the oil will spit, so you may want to use a splatter guard. Turn the cutlet over and cook the other side for another 3 minutes—hold it flat with a spatula for the last minute or so.

While the chicken is cooking, put the salad together. Squeeze one of the lemon slices over the green salad and arugula leaves and radishes, and mix everything together well. Check that the chicken is done—the juices will run clear when it is—and lift it out of the pan. Blot it briefly on paper towels and put it on a warmed serving plate. Squeeze the other slice of lemon over it, grind a little black pepper on top, and serve immediately with the salad on the side.

Tip:

▶ You could also use a turkey cutlet in this dish and substitute other spices—try a Cajun spice mix, for example. Don't use too much, though, as it can burn easily and taste bitter.

Chicken or turkey stir-fry with snow peas and green beans
Serves 1

1 small chicken breast, about
3½ oz (100 g), skin
removed, or turkey breast
of the same weight
juice of half a lemon
1 tsp light soy sauce
¼ cup (¾ oz) snow peas,
trimmed

SERVINGS		NUTRITIONAL INFO	
Protein	3½	Calories	235
Fat	1	Carbohydrate	8 g
Dairy	0	Protein	30 g
Fruit	0	Fiber	6 g
Vegetables	2½	Salt	0.8 g

½ *cup (1¾ oz) thin string*   ½-*in-square piece of fresh*
   beans, trimmed   *ginger root, finely chopped*
2 *spears broccolini*   1 *small red chili, deseeded*
4 *scallions, sliced diagonally*   *and finely chopped*
1 *garlic clove, finely chopped*   (*optional*)
                        2 *tsp canola oil*

Cut the chicken or turkey breast into ¼-by-2⅓-in strips. Put these in a bowl and add a teaspoon of the lemon juice and the soy sauce. Stir to coat, then cover the bowl with plastic wrap and put it in the refrigerator for 30 minutes.

Prepare all the vegetables: chop the snow peas and beans into strips the same length as the chicken or turkey pieces; break up the spears of broccolini and cut off any woody stems; slice the scallions diagonally and include some of the green part.

Put a nonstick wok or large nonstick frying pan on high heat, add the oil, and take the chicken or turkey strips out of the refrigerator. Using a slotted spoon, remove the meat from the marinade and put it into the wok—it should spit if the oil is hot enough, so be careful. Cook for about 3–4 minutes, stirring well until the meat begins to color, then remove the meat from the wok and set aside. Add the chopped vegetables, scallions, garlic, ginger, and chili and cook them quickly until crisp but tender; stir them around or they will stick to the pan and burn. Return the meat and any juices to the wok, add the rest of the lemon juice, and allow the chicken to heat up thoroughly, which will take another minute or two. Serve immediately.

Tangy chicken drumsticks with crudités and a harissa dip
Serves 1

2 chicken drumsticks, skin removed, about 4 oz (120 g) each

For the marinade:
2 scallions, finely chopped
3 tbsp Worcestershire sauce
splash Tabasco sauce
black pepper
½ tsp cinnamon
½ tsp ground allspice
¼ tsp ground cumin
1 tbsp cider vinegar

SERVINGS		NUTRITIONAL INFO	
Protein	5	Calories	282
Fat	0	Carbohydrate	12 g
Dairy	½	Protein	45 g
Fruit	0	Fiber	3 g
Vegetables	2½	Salt	1 g

For the crudités and dip:
3 celery sticks
3 scallions
2-in piece of cucumber
2 tbsp low-fat or fat-free Greek yogurt
½–1 tsp harissa (to taste)

Carefully remove the skin from the drumsticks. Mix all the marinade ingredients together in a small ceramic or glass dish just large enough to hold the two drumsticks. Put the drumsticks in and turn them in the marinade, then spoon some of the marinade over them. Cover with plastic wrap and refrigerate for at least 6 hours, but for no longer than 12 hours.

Preheat the oven to 375°F. Lift the chicken out of the marinade, then strain the remainder of the marinade into a small baking dish (discard the scallions left in the strainer). Add a tablespoon of water and the chicken drumsticks. Turn them over and over in the marinade and then put the baking dish in the oven. Cook for 35–40 minutes, or until the drumsticks are done, which will depend on their size. Turn them over twice during this time.

Prepare the crudités and dip just before the drumsticks are ready. Trim the celery, removing the strings with a knife, and the scallions. Peel the cucumber, cut it in half, remove the seeds, and then slice it into strips. Spoon the yogurt into a small bowl and gradually add the harissa, tasting it as you go along to make sure that you get the dip just as hot as you want it. Serve with the crudités as soon as the drumsticks are ready.

Tips:

▶ Instead of using individual spices in the marinade, you could use a teaspoon of jerk seasoning; it will taste different but be equally good. If the brand you choose has a high proportion of chili in it—they vary—don't use the Tabasco.

▶ The drumsticks can also be served cold.

"Not quite coronation chicken"
Serves 1

½ tsp garam masala

¼ tsp turmeric

2 tbsp low-fat or fat-free
    Greek yogurt

1 tbsp low-fat mayonnaise

dash of Worcestershire sauce,
    to taste

black pepper

5 oz (150 g) cooked chicken
    breast, skin and any excess
    fat removed

1 celery stick, trimmed

2 scallions, trimmed

SERVINGS		NUTRITIONAL INFO	
Protein	5	Calories	430
Fat	2	Carbohydrate	12 g
Dairy	½	Protein	56 g
Fruit	0	Fiber	3 g
Vegetables	½	Salt	1.3 g

handful of lettuce leaves,
    about 2 oz (60 g)

handful of sliced almonds,
    about ⅓ oz (10 g)

Put a nonstick frying pan on medium heat. When it is hot, spoon in the garam masala and turmeric and stir them around until they begin to smell toasted. As soon as they reach that stage, take the pan off the heat and tip the spices into a bowl.

Add the yogurt and the mayonnaise to the bowl, with a small dash of Worcestershire sauce. Stir them together, then taste; add more Worcestershire sauce if needed. Grind in some black pepper. Chop the chicken breast into chunks about ½ in square and add these to the bowl. Stir everything together, cover the bowl with plastic wrap, and refrigerate for at least an hour, preferably two.

Pull the strings from the celery stick and chop it into small pieces, then chop one scallion into diagonal slices and the other into finer pieces. Take the chicken out of the refrigerator, add the chopped celery and scallion, and stir everything together. Put the salad leaves on a serving plate and spoon the chicken salad on top; top with the almonds and serve immediately.

Grilled chicken with Asian slaw and a quick sambal

Serves 1

Juice and zest of 1 lime
½ tsp dark soy sauce
1 skinless chicken breast,
* weighing 4 oz (120 g)*
1½ tbsp shredded white cabbage
1½ oz (40 g) romaine lettuce
* leaves, roughly torn*
3 baby corns, sliced in half
* vertically*

SERVINGS		NUTRITIONAL INFO	
Protein	4	Calories	170
Fat	0	Carbohydrate	6 g
Dairy	0	Protein	30 g
Fruit	0	Fiber	3 g
Vegetables	1½	Salt	0.7 g

1 tbsp chopped cilantro

¼-in piece of ginger root,
   finely grated

For the sambal:

1 red chili, finely chopped

½ garlic clove, crushed

squeeze of lime juice

Drizzle half the lime juice and zest and the soy sauce over the chicken and set aside in the fridge for a minimum of 1 hour, up to overnight.

Heat a grill pan over medium heat. When smoking hot, add the chicken breast and grill for 4 minutes on each side. Check that the chicken is cooked by inserting a skewer into the thickest part of the meat—if the juices run clear, set the chicken breast aside. Grill for another 2–3 minutes, if necessary.

Meanwhile, toss the cabbage, lettuce, baby corn, and cilantro in the ginger and remaining lime juice and zest and set aside.

To make the sambal, crush the ingredients together in a mortar and pestle until they form a thick, homogenous paste.

Serve the chicken hot or cold with the slaw and the sambal.

Meat dishes

Grilled lamb, eggplant, and sun-dried tomato stack
Serves 1

1 tsp tomato purée

1 garlic clove, crushed

¼ tsp olive oil

¼ tsp fennel seeds, crushed in
   a mortar and pestle

SERVINGS		NUTRITIONAL INFO	
Protein	4	Calories	280
Fat	0	Carbohydrate	6 g
Dairy	0	Protein	27 g
Fruit	0	Fiber	5 g
Vegetables	1½	Salt	0.5 g

4 oz (120 g) lamb loin,
   sliced into ¼-in slices
⅓ medium eggplant,
   sliced into ¼-in slices

2 sun-dried tomatoes,
   chopped
small handful of basil leaves
½ tsp balsamic vinegar
black pepper

Mix together the tomato purée, garlic, olive oil, and fennel seeds and brush over the lamb and eggplant. Preheat a grill pan over high heat and when smoking hot, grill the lamb and eggplant slices for 1 minute each side. Remove from the pan and layer the slices up on a plate, sprinkling with the sun-dried tomato and basil. Finish by drizzling with the balsamic vinegar and seasoning with black pepper.

Harissa-roasted pork fillet with pumpkin and tomatoes
Serves 1

½ tsp caraway seeds
¼ tsp coriander seeds
½ tsp paprika
1 red chili
1 garlic clove
¼ tsp olive oil
4 oz (120 g) pork fillet, sinew
   and fatty bits sliced off
2¾ oz (80 g) pumpkin,
   chopped into ¼-in dice

SERVINGS		NUTRITIONAL INFO	
Protein	4	Calories	175
Fat	0	Carbohydrate	5 g
Dairy	0	Protein	31 g
Fruit	0	Fiber	6 g
Vegetables	2	Salt	0.2 g

1 medium tomato, sliced into
   quarters
1 tsp lemon juice
1 tbsp cilantro, chopped

Toast the caraway seeds, coriander seeds, and paprika in a small frying pan for 1 minute, until fragrant.

To make the harissa, crush the chili, garlic, toasted spices, and olive oil together in a mortar and pestle until they make a paste. Rub the harissa over the pork fillet until completely covered. Set aside in the fridge for a minimum of 2 hours, up to overnight.

Preheat the oven to 375°F.

Transfer the pork fillet to an ovenproof dish, add the pumpkin and tomatoes to the dish, and toss together so that everything is coated in a little harissa.

Roast in the oven for 15–20 minutes, until the juices of the fillet run clear when pierced with a skewer. Drizzle with the lemon juice, sprinkle with the cilantro, and serve immediately.

Lamb chops and "little dishes"

Serves 1

2 small lamb chops or cutlets
(about 4 oz/120 g)
1 tsp olive oil
¼ tsp paprika
pinch of turmeric
pinch of cayenne
handful of mint leaves,
finely chopped
2 sprigs of rosemary

SERVINGS		NUTRITIONAL INFO	
Protein	4	Calories	383
Fat	1½	Carbohydrate	7 g
Dairy	0	Protein	38 g
Fruit	0	Fiber	3 g
Vegetables	3	Salt	0.6 g

For the "little dishes":
2-in piece of cucumber
6 large green olives

handful of salad leaves,
about 2 oz (60 g)

7 cherry tomatoes, sliced   *1 tsp balsamic vinegar*
1 tsp olive oil   *½ red chili (optional)*
squeeze of lemon juice

You will need a ceramic or glass ovenproof dish. Pat the chops dry and remove any excess fat; if you are using cutlets, strip the fat from the bone.

Put the olive oil in the bottom of the ovenproof dish and add the paprika, turmeric, and cayenne, along with the chopped mint leaves and the whole rosemary sprigs. Mix everything together and then add the chops. Move them about to coat them in the oil-and-spice mix, then turn the chops over so the other side is coated with the mixture as well. Cover the dish with plastic wrap and leave it in the refrigerator for an hour.

Near the end of that time, preheat the oven to 400°F and start to prepare the "little dishes." Peel the cucumber, slice it very thinly, then set aside.

Take the plastic wrap off the ovenproof dish and put it in the oven. Cook the lamb for approximately 6 minutes, and then turn the chops over and cook for another 6 minutes, or until the lamb is done to your liking (exactly how long will depend on the thickness of the meat and personal taste).

While the lamb is cooking, finish the accompaniments. Put the olives in a little dish—rinse them first if they have been in brine. Put the salad leaves in a bowl. Scatter the sliced cherry tomatoes over the salad leaves. Dress the salad by drizzling with the olive oil, toss, then add a squeeze of lemon juice. Rinse the cucumber slices and put these in another small dish, add the balsamic vinegar, and stir. Very finely slice the red chili and scatter over the cucumber slices.

As soon as the meat is ready, lift it out of the ovenproof dish onto a serving plate. Serve surrounded by the "little dishes."

Tip

▶ If you're not fond of lamb, substitute chicken breast, but note that it will take much longer to cook, so adjust the timings accordingly. The chicken breast could also be grilled rather than roasted, as could the lamb chops.

Vegetarian mains

Quick cauliflower and okra curry with a yogurt and mint raita

Serves 1

½ tsp olive oil

2 scallions, sliced

1 garlic clove, crushed

½-in piece of ginger root, finely grated

½ tsp ground cumin seeds

½ tsp ground coriander seeds

¼ tsp garam masala

¼ tsp hot chili powder

¼ tsp black mustard seeds (optional)

4 cauliflower florets (1½ oz/40 g)

½ 14-oz can chopped tomatoes

8 small okra

1 tbsp chopped cilantro

For the raita:

3 tbsp fat-free plain yogurt

1-in piece of cucumber, peeled, coarsely grated

1 tsp finely chopped mint

SERVINGS		NUTRITIONAL INFO	
Protein	0	Calories	106
Fat	0	Carbohydrate	13 g
Dairy	1	Protein	7 g
Fruit	0	Fiber	7 g
Vegetables	2½	Salt	0.2 g

Heat the oil in a medium frying pan over medium heat. When the oil is hot, add the scallions and fry gently for 2–3 minutes, until softened and golden. Add the garlic, ginger, spices, and cauliflower and fry for another 1 or 2 minutes, until fragrant and the cauliflower is golden. Add the tomatoes and simmer for 3–4 minutes, until the sauce has thickened and reduced slightly. Add the okra and cook for another 2 minutes, until slightly softened.

Meanwhile, mix together the yogurt, cucumber, and mint to make the raita. Serve the curry sprinkled with the cilantro and the raita on the side.

Ginger, soy, and chili tofu skewers with Chinese cabbage and snow pea salad

Serves 1

4⅓ oz (125 g) firm tofu
2 tsp low-salt soy sauce
¼ tsp sesame oil
¼ tsp crushed chili flakes
½-in piece of ginger root,
 finely grated

SERVINGS		NUTRITIONAL INFO	
Protein	2½	Calories	151
Fat	0	Carbohydrate	8 g
Dairy	0	Protein	15 g
Fruit	0	Fiber	4 g
Vegetables	2	Salt	1.8 g

For the salad:
⅕ of a head of Chinese,
 cabbage, finely sliced
2¾ oz (80 g) snow peas,
 sliced in half lengthwise

For the dressing:
½ red chili, finely chopped
juice of half a lime
½ lemongrass stalk, woody
 outer layers removed and
 finely sliced

For the skewers, slice the tofu into long strips, approximately 4 in long and 1 in wide, and thread onto wooden skewers.

Transfer the skewers onto a baking pan and mix together the soy sauce, sesame oil, chili flakes, and ginger; pour over the skewers. Set aside to marinate for up to an hour, turning the skewers over occasionally to marinate evenly.

Meanwhile, mix together the chili, lime juice, and lemongrass for the dressing.

Preheat the broiler to high and broil the skewers for 1–2 minutes each side, until browned.

Toss the cabbage and snow peas in the dressing and serve with the skewers and any juices left in the broiler pan.

Italian bean stew

Serves 2

7½ oz (1 x 227 g) can
  whole or chopped plum
  tomatoes
1 tsp olive oil
1 leek, trimmed
  and chopped
1 celery stick, chopped
2 garlic cloves, chopped
1 tsp dried mixed herbs,
  Italian if available
5½ oz (160 g) finely chopped
  curly kale or savoy
  cabbage leaves

4 oz (120 g) frozen soybeans
black pepper

SERVINGS		NUTRITIONAL INFO	
Protein	1	Calories	172
Fat	0	Carbohydrate	11 g
Dairy	0	Protein	14 g
Fruit	0	Fiber	9 g
Vegetables	2½	Salt	0.2 g

Drain the can of tomatoes over a bowl and set aside the juice. Put a pan over a medium heat and add the oil. Once hot, add the leek and celery and cook them gently, stirring, until they start to soften; don't let them burn. Add the garlic, stir it in, and cook for another 1 minute. Then add the tomatoes, breaking them up as you stir them in, and a sprinkling of the mixed herbs.

Cook very gently for another 8–10 minutes, stirring regularly, until everything is really tender. Keep an eye on the pan, and if it looks as though the mixture is sticking to the bottom, lower the temperature and add a splash of water.

Now add the chopped kale or cabbage and the juice from the tomatoes, and simmer for 15 minutes or so, until the kale is thoroughly cooked; again, if it looks as though the liquid may be evaporating too quickly, add a little more water. Finally, add the frozen soybeans and cook the stew for 7–8 minutes, or until the beans are soft but not mushy; adjust the heat if necessary so that you end up with a stew and not a soup (see the tip below). Check the seasoning, add a little black pepper, and serve immediately.

Tip:

▶ This recipe also makes a great thick and chunky soup—just rinse out the tomato can with water and add that water to the pan to increase the amount of liquid.

▶ Stew or soup, this dish freezes beautifully, and a little grated cheese (such as Edam) is delicious on top.

Mint, feta, and soybean salad
Serves 1

2 oz (60 g) frozen soybeans or fresh edamame
1 tsp olive oil
½ tsp balsamic vinegar

¼ tsp Dijon or whole grain mustard
2 celery sticks, strings removed and finely chopped

6 scallions, chopped

½-in piece of cucumber

2 sprigs of fresh mint,
leaves removed

1 oz (30 g) feta cheese

SERVINGS		NUTRITIONAL INFO	
Protein	1	Calories	220
Fat	½	Carbohydrate	8 g
Dairy	1	Protein	16 g
Fruit	0	Fiber	7 g
Vegetables	2½	Salt	1.4 g

To serve:

handful of lettuce leaves,   *black pepper*
about 2 oz (60 g)

Bring a pot of water to a boil and add the frozen soybeans. Return to a boil, then lower the heat and simmer until tender, about 7–8 minutes. Test the beans as they cook and be careful not to overdo them—not only do they get mushy, they also lose their attractive bright-green color. Cook fresh edamame for a shorter time, until warm and tender. Once cooked, drain and set aside.

Put the oil, vinegar, and mustard in a large bowl and beat them together until the mustard is dissolved, then add the warm beans. Stir them well and set the bowl aside.

Prepare the rest of the ingredients: chop the celery and scallions; partly peel the cucumber along its length, making stripes, then cut in half lengthwise; remove the seeds and cut the halves across into semicircles. Take the mint leaves, roll them up, and chop them into fine strips. Put all the chopped vegetables and the mint into the bowl with the soybeans and stir everything together well.

Rinse the feta under cool running water to get rid of any excess brine.

Put the lettuce leaves on a serving plate and top with the fresh bean salad. Then crumble the feta over the top and add a generous amount of black pepper. Serve immediately.

Baked eggs, Tunisian style
Serves 1

1 tsp olive oil
½ green bell pepper, deseeded
   and chopped
½ leek, sliced into rings
1 garlic clove, finely
   chopped
½ yellow squash
   (zucchini if unavailable),
   sliced into rings
1 medium tomato, deseeded
   and chopped
½ tsp paprika

¼–½ tsp cayenne pepper, to
   taste
dash of wine vinegar
black pepper
2 eggs

SERVINGS		NUTRITIONAL INFO	
Protein	2	Calories	265
Fat	½	Carbohydrate	9 g
Dairy	0	Protein	19 g
Fruit	0	Fiber	6 g
Vegetables	3½	Salt	0.5 g

Preheat the oven to 400°F.

Heat the oil in a small pan over medium heat, then add the bell pepper and cook gently for about 2 minutes. Then add the leek and garlic and cook the mixture gently for another 5–10 minutes, stirring so that it doesn't burn (cover the pan if you wish, but don't forget to check it). Then add the squash, tomato, paprika, and cayenne pepper. Add a dash of vinegar and plenty of black pepper and cook the mixture for another 5 minutes. Meanwhile, find a small ovenproof dish that can also be taken to the table and warm it in the oven.

Spoon the vegetable mixture into the warmed ovenproof dish and make two depressions in the surface of the mixture with the back of a ladle or a wooden spoon; don't press right through to the surface of the dish. (If there isn't room for two separate depressions, make a single larger one in the middle.) Break the eggs, one by one, into a cup and slide them into these dips. Put the dish into the oven and bake until the eggs are just set—the yolks should be runny and the whites set—which will take about 8 minutes. Serve immediately, straight from the dish.

Stuffed portobello mushrooms

Serves 1

2 large portobello mushrooms, about 5 oz (150 g) in total, wiped

3½ oz (½ cups) fresh spinach leaves, washed, stringy stalks removed, and chopped

4 walnut halves (optional), roughly chopped

black pepper

1 oz (30 g) low-fat mozzarella

1 tsp good-quality pesto

scant tsp balsamic vinegar

To serve:

handful of salad leaves, about 2 oz (60 g)

SERVINGS		NUTRITIONAL INFO	
Protein	0	Calories	234
Fat	2	Carbohydrate	3 g
Dairy	1	Protein	15 g
Fruit	0	Fiber	5 g
Vegetables	4	Salt	0.6 g

Preheat the oven to 400°F. Use a small ovenproof dish, just big enough to hold the mushrooms without their tipping over, and line it with foil. Wipe the mushrooms (only peel them if necessary). Trim the stalks so that the interior is flattish and put the caps in the dish, stalk side uppermost. Put the dish in the oven and bake the mushrooms for 15 minutes.

Toward the end of this time, put the washed and prepared spinach in a pan over medium heat; there's no need to add any extra water. Wilt it down until it is hugely reduced in volume, stirring regularly to make sure it doesn't stick—this will only take about 2–3 minutes.

Drain the spinach well, pressing it down in the strainer to get as much liquid out as possible. Empty the spinach out onto a chopping board and chop it again, even more finely. Add the roughly chopped walnuts to the spinach, along with plenty of black pepper, and mix them in. Cut the mozzarella into small pieces and set aside.

Take the mushrooms out of the oven. Carefully spread a teaspoon of pesto over each one, then divide the spinach-and-walnut mixture between them. Scatter the pieces of mozzarella on top and return the dish to the oven for 5–6 minutes, until the mozzarella is beginning to spread and color up.

Put the stuffed mushrooms on a plate and drizzle a little balsamic vinegar across the surface. Serve immediately, accompanied by a side dish of salad leaves

Tip:

▶ Buy a good-quality pesto; it's worth it. Less expensive varieties often contain cheaper oils than pure olive oil, and cashews rather than pine nuts. Some are even padded out with potato flakes and sugar, so check the ingredients list carefully.

Roasted vegetables with broiled halloumi
Serves 1

¼ of a small acorn squash,
about 2¾ oz
½ small eggplant, about
2¾ oz (80 g)
½ green bell pepper
1 tsp olive oil
½ large zucchini, chopped

SERVINGS		NUTRITIONAL INFO	
Protein	0	Calories	233
Fat	0	Carbohydrate	6 g
Dairy	1½	Protein	15 g
Fruit	0	Fiber	4 g
Vegetables	4	Salt	0.8 g

For the halloumi:
1¾ oz (50 g) low-fat or light
halloumi, sliced
pinch or two of dried thyme
or oregano

½ tsp olive oil
handful of fresh oregano
(optional)

Preheat the oven to 400°F. Peel the acorn squash and discard any seeds and stringy bits. Cut the flesh into chunks of about ½ in (you should have about 3 heaping tablespoons). Chop the eggplant and pepper into pieces of about the same size. Put the teaspoon of olive oil into a small roasting pan or ovenproof dish and pop it in the oven to warm through. When it is warm, tip the dish so that the oil runs across it, then add the acorn squash, eggplant, and bell pepper. Spread them out, turning each piece in the oil, and put the dish back in the oven for 15 minutes. Then stir the vegetables again and add the chopped zucchini. Return the dish to the oven for another 10 minutes and check the vegetables for softness—they may take another 5 minutes or so, depending on the squash used.

When the vegetables are nearly ready, prepare the halloumi. If you have a separate broiler and oven, preheat the broiler, brush the slices with the oil, and rub the herbs into them. Pop the slices on foil and broil both sides.

If your oven and broiler are combined, preheat a small non-stick frying pan. Sprinkle both sides of the halloumi slices with a little dried thyme or oregano and add the half teaspoon of olive oil to the pan. When the pan is hot, fry the halloumi quickly for about 1 minute on each side.

Put the vegetables on a serving plate and carefully lift and place the halloumi beside them. Scatter the fresh oregano over everything, if using, and serve immediately.

Tip:

▶ If you can't find low-fat halloumi, you can use low-fat mozzarella instead, but treat it a little differently. Once the roasted vegetables are tender, scatter 1¾ oz (50 g) of chopped mozzarella on top; pop the dish under a hot grill until the mozzarella has melted and serve immediately.

Fluffy omelette with scallions

Serves 1

2 eggs
black pepper
a little sunflower spread
3 large scallions, trimmed
    and finely chopped
⅓ oz (10 g) low-fat
    cheddar cheese, grated

SERVINGS		NUTRITIONAL INFO	
Protein	2	Calories	258
Fat	0	Carbohydrate	1 g
Dairy	½	Protein	21 g
Fruit	0	Fiber	1 g
Vegetables	1½	Salt	0.7 g

To garnish:
handful of watercress, about 2¾ oz (80 g)

Carefully separate the eggs into yolks and whites and put them in two separate bowls. Beat the yolks, adding a little black pepper to them. Whisk the whites—an electric whisk makes this easier—until they stand in soft peaks. Then carefully fold them into the beaten yolks, bit by bit.

   Melt the sunflower spread in a small nonstick frying pan over low to medium heat. Pour in the egg mixture and level the surface off with an offset spatula or similar flat utensil. Then scatter the scallions over it and finally add the grated cheese. Cook the omelette for 4–5 minutes, by which time the top should be fluffy and warm and the underside (when you lift it up slightly with your spatula) golden brown. Slide the omelette onto a serving plate, allowing it to fold over slightly as you do so, and garnish with the watercress. Serve immediately.

"Almost a céleri rémoulade"
Serves 1

5 oz (150 g) untrimmed
*   celeriac*
3 celery sticks

For the dressing:
½ tsp Dijon mustard
1 tbsp low-fat mayonnaise
1 tsp capers
black pepper

SERVINGS		NUTRITIONAL INFO	
Protein	0	Calories	148
Fat	1	Carbohydrate	9 g
Dairy	0	Protein	4 g
Fruit	0	Fiber	5 g
Vegetables	4	Salt	1.6 g

To serve:
handful of iceberg lettuce leaves, about 2¾ oz (80 g)

Make the dressing first. Put the mustard and the mayonnaise in a large bowl. Rinse the capers (they are generally sold in brine), chop them roughly, then add them to the bowl as well. Stir everything together, adding black pepper to taste.

Put a pot of water on to boil. Trim the celeriac and cut into thin pieces about 1 in long wherever possible, then cut these pieces into fine matchsticks.

Once all the celeriac is ready, carefully slide the strips into the pot of rapidly boiling water. Return the water to the boil and cook the celeriac for just 1 minute, then drain it in a strainer. Rinse it immediately under cold water and shake it well to dry it thoroughly (if necessary, pat dry in a clean dish towel or with paper towels).

While it is drying off, prepare the celery sticks. Pull off any strings, then slice each in two down the length of the sticks and then slice across very finely. Put these into the bowl with the dressing and then add the cool celeriac. Mix everything carefully, ensuring all the celeriac and celery is coated with the dressing, then cover the bowl with plastic wrap and refrigerate for an hour.

Serve with scoops made from iceberg lettuce leaves.

Tip:
▶ This is also good served with a chicken breast or a salmon fillet (see page 275, "Baked chicken with rosemary," or page 199, "Salmon parcels with aromatic salad," for ideas).

Oriental vegetable stir-fry with marinated tofu and cashews

Serves 1

5 oz (150 g) firm tofu

juice of 1 lemon

1 tsp light soy sauce

1 small pak choi
   or half a large
   one, trimmed (about
   2 oz/60 g)

6 scallions

1 large garlic clove, finely
   chopped

¼–½-in piece of fresh
   ginger root, finely
   chopped

2 tsp canola or other
   neutral-tasting vegetable
   oil

2 handfuls of bean sprouts—
   about 4 tbsp

1 tbsp cashew nuts

SERVINGS		NUTRITIONAL INFO	
Protein	2½	Calories	286
Fat	1½	Carbohydrate	12 g
Dairy	0	Protein	19 g
Fruit	0	Fiber	6 g
Vegetables	2½	Salt	0.6 g

Carefully cut the block of tofu into slices about ¼ in thick. Put the lemon juice and soy sauce in a dish and blend them together. Spread out a double thickness of paper towels, then gently lift the first slice of tofu onto the towel, fold the towel over, and lightly press down on the tofu to blot it. Peel the towel back and then carefully lift the tofu slice into the dish with the marinade. Repeat with the other slices and then spoon a little of the marinade over the tofu pieces. Cover and leave for 10 minutes, then very carefully turn the slices over. Leave for another 10 minutes.

Take the pak choi and slice the leaf part into very fine strips, then push to one side while you cut the stems into broader pieces. Chop the scallions diagonally across, including some of the green part. Set these aside with the chopped garlic and ginger.

Heat the oil in a nonstick wok or large nonstick frying pan until it is hot. Get some more paper towels, lift the tofu out of the marinade, and blot it as before. Cut each slice in half, making rough squares, and gently lower them into the wok. Cook for 3 minutes, and then turn them over carefully. Take the wok off the heat while doing this, so the remaining ones don't overcook, then return the wok to the heat and cook the other sides. Have a plate ready, and lift the pieces of tofu onto the plate with a spatula, again doing so with the wok off the heat.

Return the wok to the heat—enough oil should have remained in it—and add the scallions, pak choi stems, garlic, and ginger. Cook and stir these for 3 minutes, then add the bean sprouts and the pak choi leaf strips. Stir briefly, then add a tablespoon of the marinade and cook it off, stirring. Add the cashew nuts and stir the vegetables around, then carefully replace the tofu. Cook without stirring for a few more seconds and then transfer the stir-fry to a warm plate. Serve immediately.

Tip:

▶ Tofu can be difficult to handle, but it is worth it; not only is it highly nutritious, it takes up flavors beautifully.

Cauliflower and mushroom curry with yogurt
Serves 2

1 small cauliflower (about 7 oz/200 g)
8 oz (250 g) mushrooms
½ tsp cayenne pepper

½ tsp ground coriander
½ tsp ground cumin
½ tsp turmeric
½ tsp ground black pepper

2 tsp canola or other neutral-
tasting vegetable oil
1 cup (8 fl oz) boiling water
2 heaping tbsp plain yogurt
handful of sliced almonds,
or a handful of cilantro
leaves, chopped

SERVINGS		NUTRITIONAL INFO	
Protein	0	Calories	153
Fat	1	Carbohydrate	8 g
Dairy	1	Protein	10 g
Fruit	0	Fiber	5 g
Vegetables	3	Salt	0.1 g

Trim the cauliflower and break the florets into pieces no larger than ½ in; clean and slice the mushrooms. Set the vegetables aside. Put all the spices and the black pepper in a small bowl and mix them together.

Put the oil in a large pan and warm it up over medium heat. Once it is hot, add the spices, stir, and sauté for 1 minute. Add the mushrooms and the cauliflower florets and stir for another minute—don't stop stirring, or they could stick to the pan.

Add the boiling water to the vegetables and bring the pan to a simmer. Cover and cook for 10 minutes, then lift the lid and check on the amount of liquid remaining. If there is still a large amount of liquid, leave the lid off for another 5 minutes, or until the pieces of cauliflower are tender; otherwise replace the lid, but keep checking. After 5 minutes the sauce should be reduced to almost nothing; increase the heat briefly, if necessary, to reduce it further, but don't stir the curry too much or the florets may break up.

As soon as the cauliflower is tender and the sauce is much reduced, spoon the curry into serving bowls. Top each helping with a generous spoonful of yogurt and top with a few almonds or some cilantro leaves. Serve immediately.

Green vegetable gratin

Serves 1

1 medium tomato, chopped
½ medium zucchini
(about 1¾ oz/50 g)
½ tsp olive oil
½ small leek, trimmed
and chopped
1 garlic clove, finely
chopped
1¾ oz (50 g) frozen soybeans
several florets of broccoli
(about 2¾ oz/80 g)

SERVINGS		NUTRITIONAL INFO	
Protein	1	Calories	262
Fat	0	Carbohydrate	11 g
Dairy	1	Protein	22 g
Fruit	0	Fiber	10 g
Vegetables	4	Salt	0.8 g

1 oz (30 g) Edam cheese,
grated
black pepper

Preheat the oven to 350°F. You will need a small ovenproof dish—it should be about 2 in deep.

Put the chopped tomato in a small nonstick pan with a tablespoon of water. Bring to a simmer and keep an eye on it—there isn't much liquid, so you may need to add more water to prevent it from sticking to the bottom of the pan (this will depend on how juicy the tomato is). While the tomato is cooking, chop the zucchini across into round slices.

When the tomato is soft, remove from the heat and pour into a strainer over a small bowl, pressing through firmly; discard the pulp.

Rinse the tomato pan, add the olive oil, and return the pan to the heat. Add the leek and garlic and stir in the hot oil for a minute or so, until they just begin to take on color. Then pour the strained tomato sauce back into the pan and cook it until it has reduced by half, about 1 minute. Meanwhile, put a pot of water on to boil. As soon as the water is boiling, add the frozen soybeans and cook them for 1 minute. Then add the broccoli florets and cook for another 2 minutes. Finally, add all the zucchini rounds and cook everything for 1 minute more.

Drain the vegetables well. Carefully remove the zucchini rounds and set these to one side, then put the rest of the vegetables in the ovenproof dish. Pour the tomato and leek sauce over them—don't worry that there doesn't seem to be much—and then place the zucchini circles over the top, covering the vegetables. Press the zucchini down gently but firmly. Now scatter the grated Edam over the top and add plenty of black pepper. Put the dish in the preheated oven and bake for 30 minutes, until the top is golden.

Remove the gratin from the oven and carefully lift the cheesy zucchini topping onto one side of a serving plate. Using a slotted spoon, lift the vegetables out and arrange these beside the topping, then spoon a little of the tomato-flavored liquid on top. Serve immediately.

Tip:

▶ This is a very flexible recipe and invites variations. Still using half a zucchini cut into rounds for the topping, add several good handfuls of dark-green kale, roughly chopped. Blanch the kale very briefly in the boiling water just before you drain it.

Refreshing drinks

Ayran yogurt drink
Serves 1

3½ oz (100 g) plain yogurt
chilled water, still or
*   sparkling, or soda water*

SERVINGS		NUTRITIONAL INFO	
Protein	0	Calories	79
Fat	0	Carbohydrate	8 g
Dairy	1½	Protein	6 g
Fruit	0	Fiber	0 g
Vegetables	0	Salt	0.2 g

Put the yogurt in a tall glass and fill the glass with water. Whisk the two together until thoroughly combined and drink immediately.

Green mint tea
Serves 1

You can have unlimited tea. Calorie-free.

large handful of fresh mint
1 green tea bag

Strip the mint leaves from the stems. Warm a teapot, pitcher, or bowl with boiling water, discard the water, and then add the mint leaves. Add just enough boiling water to cover the leaves, swirl it around the pot, then pour out the water, retaining the leaves. Next add the tea bag and refill the pot with boiling water. Let infuse for 10 minutes before drinking.

Lemon and ginger tea

Serves 1

You can have unlimited
tea. Calorie-free.

half lemon

½-in-square piece of fresh ginger root, peeled

Cut a slice off the lemon, then squeeze the juice from the rest of the fruit into a heatproof glass or mug. Grate as much of the ginger root as possible into the glass. Top with boiling water, add the slice of lemon, stir well, and leave for 5 minutes before drinking.

Tips:

▶ For a savory drink, dissolve ¼ teaspoon of yeast extract in hot water.

▶ Make lemon balm tea in the same way as the mint tea on page 243, but leave out the tea bag.

▶ Make chili "tea" if you're feeling brave or have a cold coming on: add a small amount of chopped chili to the lemon-and-ginger drink above, but pass it through a strainer and into a clean glass before drinking.

▶ Make a cool mint tea as on page 243, but leave out the tea bag and add double the amount of mint. Allow it to cool, then add some of it (to taste) to a glass and top up with sparkling water. Add ice cubes.

10

recipes for unrestricted days

Recipes for the five unrestricted days

Zucchini frittata (V)	297
Eggplant curry with chickpeas, rice, and a mango raita (V)	298
Sweets and desserts	
Lemon and blueberry yogurt cake (V)	300
Yogurt ice cream with raspberries (V)	301
Individual lemon and honey cheesecakes (V)	302
Crunchy blackberry and apple crumble (V)	303
Crêpes (V)	304
Apricot and apple fruit salad (V)	306
Baked nectarines stuffed with nuts (V)	306
Chocolate and orange mousse (V)	307
Prune delight (V)	309
Apple fool with heather honey (V)	310
Hosaf—Turkish dried fruit salad (V)	311

Breakfast

Oatmeal with dried fruit
Serves 1

2 heaping tbsp steel-cut oats
(about 1½ oz/40 g)
1 level tsp golden raisins
1 cup (8 fl oz) water or
1% or fat-free milk
2 dried apricots, chopped

SERVINGS		NUTRITIONAL INFO	
If using fat-free milk			
Carbohydrate	2	Calories	286
Protein	0	Carbohydrate	53 g
Fat	0	Protein	13 g
Dairy	1	Fiber	5 g
Fruit	1	Salt	0.3 g
Vegetables	0		

Put the oats and the raisins into a small nonstick pan and add the water or milk. Put the pan on a medium heat and bring it to a simmer. Cook for about 10 minutes, stirring frequently to prevent the porridge from sticking.

By now the oatmeal should be thickening and bubbling well. Stir as it continues to thicken for another few minutes, or until it reaches the consistency you like. Pour into a bowl and scatter the chopped apricots on top. Serve immediately.

Tips:

▶ As an alternative, add 2 chopped almonds to the apricots.

▶ If you prefer your oatmeal sweeter, stir in 1 teaspoon of clear honey.

Classic muesli
Serves 2

2¾ oz (80 g) rolled oats
4 dried apricots, chopped
4 tbsp unsweetened apple
  juice
1 sweet apple, unpeeled
2 tbsp low-fat plain yogurt
6 Brazil nuts, chopped
2 tsp clear honey (optional)

SERVINGS		NUTRITIONAL INFO	
Without honey			
Carbohydrate	2	Calories	283
Protein	0	Carbohydrate	45 g
Fat	1	Protein	8 g
Dairy	½	Fiber	6 g
Fruit	1	Salt	0.1 g
Vegetables	0		

The evening before you want to eat the muesli, put the oats, chopped apricots, and apple juice in a bowl. Stir, cover, and leave overnight.

The following morning, grate in the apple and stir well. Add the yogurt to the mixture and stir that in too. Heat a dry frying pan; when hot, add the chopped nuts, stirring them until they begin to color. Divide the muesli into two serving bowls and sprinkle with the toasted nuts. Drizzle the honey over these, if you wish.

Soups

Zucchini soup with basil and a tomato salsa
Serves 4

2 tsp olive oil
2 medium onions, peeled and chopped
2 lb 4 oz (1 kg) zucchini, trimmed and roughly chopped

4 garlic cloves, crushed

1 quart (32 fl oz) low-salt
vegetable stock

2 medium tomatoes

handful of basil leaves

black pepper

SERVINGS		NUTRITIONAL INFO	
Carbohydrate	0	Calories	146
Protein	0	Carbohydrate	17 g
Fat	0	Protein	9 g
Dairy	½	Fiber	5 g
Fruit	0	Salt	1 g
Vegetables	4		

To serve:

4 tbsp low-fat Greek yogurt

Put the olive oil in a nonstick pot over medium heat and add the onions. Cook gently, stirring so they don't stick to the bottom of the pan, for about 5 minutes, until beginning to soften. Then add the zucchini and garlic and stir these into the softened onions. Cook for about 2 minutes and add the stock, then increase the heat and bring the soup to a simmer. Cook for about 10 minutes, or until the zucchini is soft.

Make the salsa while the soup is cooking. Chop the tomatoes finely and put them in a small dish or bowl. Tear some of the basil leaves and add to the dish with a good twist of black pepper; stir everything together. Set aside while you finish the soup.

When the soup is ready, remove the pot from the heat and allow the soup to cool a little. Blend until smooth, using either a handheld blender or a blender. If you're using a blender, put the soup back into the pot and gently reheat it. Tear up the remaining basil leaves, add them to the pot, then pour the soup into serving bowls. Divide the tomato salsa among the bowls, scattering it in the center of each bowl, and top each with a swirl of Greek yogurt. Serve immediately.

Tips:

▶ If you like bread with your soup, choose a whole grain variety instead of white.

▶ This recipe is suitable for making in larger batches and freezing. If freezing, don't add the salsa!

Lentil soup with spinach and a touch of lemon
Serves 4

½ cup (4 oz/125 g) green lentils

3 cups (8 oz) fresh spinach leaves

1 tsp olive oil

1 medium onion, chopped

1 garlic clove, finely chopped

1 tsp tomato purée

1¼–1½ pints (750–850 ml) low-salt vegetable stock

juice of half a small lemon

black pepper

SERVINGS		NUTRITIONAL INFO	
Carbohydrate	0	Calories	138
Protein	1½	Carbohydrate	20 g
Fat	0	Protein	10 g
Dairy	0	Fiber	6 g
Fruit	0	Salt	1.1 g
Vegetables	1		

Rinse the lentils in a strainer under running water. Put them in a pot, cover with water, and cook over medium heat for 15–20 minutes, or until they begin to soften. Then drain and rinse them once more. Set aside.

Wash the spinach leaves and remove any really stringy stalks; chop the leaves and tender stalks. Heat the olive oil in a pot and add the chopped onion. Cook gently for 10 minutes, or until the onion is very soft but not burning, then add the garlic. Cook for 1 minute more, then stir in the lentils.

Add the wet spinach leaves, plus any chopped stalks to the pot; stir these in. Mix the tomato purée with the stock and add enough of the liquid to the pot to cover the spinach leaves and lentils. Cook for 5 minutes, then add the lemon juice and cook for another 5 minutes (the short cooking time should preserve the vivid green color of the spinach).

Test that the onions and lentils are really soft and remove the pan from the heat. Allow the soup to cool a little and then blend until it is almost smooth using either a handheld blender or a blender. If you're using a blender, put the soup back into the pot and gently reheat. Taste for seasoning, adding a little black pepper if you wish, and serve.

Tip:
▶ This recipe is suitable for making into larger batches and freezing.

Creamy mushroom soup
Serves 2

2 tsp canola or other
   vegetable oil
2 medium onions, chopped
1 lb 4 oz (600 g) large flat or
   field mushrooms
small pinch cayenne pepper
3 cups (24 oz) low-salt
   vegetable stock
1 cup (8 oz) 1% or fat-free
   milk

SERVINGS		NUTRITIONAL INFO	
Carbohydrate	0	Calories	188
Protein	0	Carbohydrate	20 g
Fat	½	Protein	12 g
Dairy	1	Fiber	6 g
Fruit	0	Salt	1.1 g
Vegetables	5		

sprig of thyme or a pinch of
   dried mixed herbs
black pepper

To serve:
3 tablespoons (1½ oz/40 g) low-fat or fat-free plain Greek
   yogurt

Heat the oil in a large pot over medium heat. Add the onions and cook gently, stirring, for about 5–10 minutes, until soft but not brown. While the onions are cooking, brush any dirt from the mushrooms (only peel them if necessary) and trim the ends off the stalks. Chop the mushrooms into chunks.

Add the cayenne pepper to the pot and stir for a few seconds before adding the mushroom pieces. Stir these for about another 2 minutes, being careful not to let them burn. Add the stock and milk. Strip the leaves from the thyme sprig into the pot or stir in the dried mixed herbs. Simmer the soup for about 20 minutes, then check for seasoning and add black pepper to taste.

Allow the soup to cool slightly, then blend it roughly using either a handheld blender or a blender—it shouldn't be too smooth. Add some more water if necessary, then return the soup to the pot (if using a blender) and reheat. Serve it with 2 teaspoons of Greek yogurt swirled into each bowl.

Tips:

▶ For a chunkier soup, blend only half the soup and then put it back into the pot with the unblended half.

▶ For a more intense flavor, use a selection of mushrooms, such as cremini, shiitake, or porcini.

▶ This recipe is suitable for making in larger batches and freezing.

Roasted red bell pepper soup

Serves 4

4 red bell peppers
2 tsp olive oil
1 medium onion, chopped
2 garlic cloves, finely chopped
3–4 cups (900 ml–1 liter)
*   low-salt vegetable stock*
14 oz (1 x 400 g) can of
*   cannellini beans, drained*
*   and rinsed*

SERVINGS		NUTRITIONAL INFO	
Carbohydrate	0	Calories	147
Protein	1	Carbohydrate	24 g
Fat	0	Protein	7 g
Dairy	0	Fiber	8 g
Fruit	0	Salt	0.9 g
Vegetables	2		

Preheat the broiler. Cut the peppers in half and remove the seeds. Put the oil in a small bowl and lightly brush some on the skin side of the peppers. Put the pepper halves on a baking pan, skin side uppermost. Place the pan under the hot broiler. Leave the peppers there until the skins begin to blister and turn black— this can take up to 20 minutes, depending on the heat of the broiler.

Take the baking pan out and cover the peppers with a dish towel. Leave them for 10 minutes, or until they are cool enough to handle, then gently peel the skin off the flesh. Discard the skins and chop the flesh; set to one side.

Put the remaining olive oil in a large pot. Add the onion and cook gently for 7–8 minutes, then add the garlic and cook for another 2–3 minutes. Stir the mixture so that it doesn't stick to the bottom of the pan (if it looks like it's doing so, add a couple of spoonfuls of stock and cool them off). Then add the chopped peppers and the cannellini beans and stir. Add enough stock to cover the peppers and beans; simmer for 15 minutes, then take the pan off the heat.

Allow the soup to cool a little, then blend until mostly smooth, using either a handheld blender or a blender. If using a blender, return the soup to the pot and reheat gently. Check for seasoning and serve.

Tips:

▶ If you'd like a nonvegetarian soup, add some chopped cooked chicken breast to the peppers and beans after they have cooked in the stock for 10 minutes. And don't blend the soup—serve it as a chunky soup instead.

▶ This recipe is suitable for making in larger batches and freezing.

Salads and light bites

Horiatiki salata—Greek salad

Serves 2

1 small romaine heart
4 large ripe tomatoes
½ cucumber, about 6 oz (180 g)
1 small red onion or
   6 scallions
1 tbsp olive oil
1 tsp balsamic vinegar
3½ oz (100 g) feta cheese

SERVINGS		NUTRITIONAL INFO	
Carbohydrate	0	Calories	265
Protein	0	Carbohydrate	13 g
Fat	2	Protein	11 g
Dairy	1½	Fiber	6 g
Fruit	0	Salt	2.1 g
Vegetables	4		

20 black olives, pitted and sliced
black pepper

Wash the lettuce leaves, tear them up, and divide them between two serving plates or bowls.

Chop the tomatoes and put them in a bowl. Cut the cucumber in half lengthwise, then chop it up and add to the tomatoes. Then peel the onion, halve it, and slice it finely (if using scallions, chop finely). Add the onion to the bowl.

Put the oil and vinegar into a small screw-top jar (a clean jam jar, for instance). Put the lid on securely, then shake to make a dressing. Pour this dressing over the tomatoes, cucumber, and onion and stir everything to combine.

Remove the feta from its packaging and rinse it under running water, then pat dry with paper towels. On a plate, cut the feta into small cubes—some brands will crumble and others will require cutting. Slide the feta into the bowl with the tomatoes. Give this mixture a final, very gentle stir and spoon it over the salad leaves. Scatter the olives over the salad, add some black pepper, and serve.

White bean salad with hard-boiled eggs

Serves 2

2 eggs
14 oz (½ x 400 g) can
   cannellini beans
½ 14 oz-can black-eyed
   beans
1 medium onion, quartered
1 bay leaf
juice of half a lemon
1 tbsp olive oil
3 celery sticks, chopped
large handful of flat-leaf
   parsley, chopped

1 small head romaine lettuce,
   leaves separated
black pepper
10 black olives, pitted and
   halved

SERVINGS		NUTRITIONAL INFO	
Carbohydrate	0	Calories	326
Protein	3	Carbohydrate	30 g
Fat	1	Protein	19 g
Dairy	0	Fiber	12 g
Fruit	0	Salt	0.5 g
Vegetables	1½		

Put the eggs in a pan of water and bring to the boil. Cook for 10 minutes, then cool rapidly under cold running water. Put them in a bowl of ice water and set aside in a cool place.

Drain the cans of beans into a large sieve and rinse them thoroughly. Put the rinsed beans in a large pan over medium to high heat, add the onion and bay leaf, and then cover them with fresh water. Bring the beans to a good rolling simmer and cook for 5 minutes, then drain them well.

Allow the beans to cool a little until they are no longer hot, but still warm; remove the bay leaf and the pieces of onion. Discard the bay leaf, but finely slice two of the onion quarters (or use all if you wish) and put them back into the beans.

In a large bowl, mix together the lemon juice, olive oil, and chopped celery and parsley. Then add the warm beans and onion, and stir everything well. Cover the beans and leave them to absorb the flavors for 30 minutes.

Wash the lettuce leaves, tear them up, and divide between two serving plates. Check the flavor of the beans and add black pepper to taste, then stir once more before dividing between the two plates. Peel the hard-boiled eggs and cut these into quarters. Decorate the salad with the eggs and the olives and serve.

A pair of potato salads
Serves 2

8 oz (250 g) new potatoes, in their skins
2 tsp balsamic vinegar
black pepper
½ cup (3½ oz) low-fat plain yogurt
2 tsp Dijon mustard

Nonvegetarian salad:
1 small red onion, sliced into
  rings
7 oz smoked mackerel or
  trout
squeeze of lemon juice
½–1 tsp horseradish sauce
  (to taste and optional)

SERVINGS		NUTRITIONAL INFO	
Carbohydrate	1	Calories	501
Protein	3½	Carbohydrate	28 g
Fat	0	Protein	25 g
Dairy	½	Fiber	3 g
Fruit	0	Salt	2.7 g
Vegetables	½		

Vegetarian salad:
6 scallions, chopped
1 ripe avocado, halved and
  pit removed
¼ cucumber, peeled, deseeded,
  and finely chopped
2 hard-boiled eggs

SERVINGS		NUTRITIONAL INFO	
Carbohydrate	1	Calories	371
Protein	1	Carbohydrate	29 g
Fat	2	Protein	15 g
Dairy	½	Fiber	7 g
Fruit	0	Salt	1 g
Vegetables	1½		

To serve:
black pepper
small handful of salad leaves, about 1 oz (30 g)

Chop the new potatoes into pieces no larger than ½ in and put them in a pot of cold water. Bring the pot to a boil, cover, and cook the potatoes until they are just soft. Drain and put them in a bowl with the balsamic vinegar and some black pepper. Turn the potatoes over carefully with a wooden spoon, then add the yogurt and mustard and stir the potatoes once more. They should still be quite warm and will absorb the flavors much better than if they were cold.

For the nonvegetarian version, add the red onion to the potatoes and stir it in. Carefully shred the smoked fish into medium-size pieces, removing any bones and skin, and squeeze over a little lemon juice. Put this in with the warm potatoes and the horseradish, if using, and mix everything together well.

For the vegetarian version, add the scallions to the potatoes. Slice through the flesh of the avocado lengthwise and across, just to the skin, but not through it, and then bend the avocado back in on itself. The chunks will either pop out by themselves or will be easy to remove. Add them to the potatoes along with the cucumber, and very gently mix them in.

Whichever version, check the seasoning and add pepper to taste. Put some salad leaves on serving plates, and divide the potato salad between them (the smoked mackerel salad is particularly good slightly warm). For the vegetarian version, peel the hard-boiled eggs and chop them finely, then scatter over the top of the salad.

Warm beet and feta salad

Serves 2

10–12 small to medium beets, uncooked (about 5 oz/150 g)
1 bag of mixed salad leaves, about 4 oz (120 g)
3½ oz (100 g) feta cheese
1 small red onion, finely sliced
1 tsp olive oil
1 tsp lemon juice
leaves from small sprig of thyme
black pepper

SERVINGS		NUTRITIONAL INFO	
Carbohydrate	0	Calories	204
Protein	0	Carbohydrate	12 g
Fat	½	Protein	10 g
Dairy	1½	Fiber	4 g
Fruit	0	Salt	2 g
Vegetables	2		

Preheat the oven to 400°F. Gently clean the raw beets but don't scrub, peel, or top and tail them; just trim off the leaves, leaving about ¼ in of stalk. Tear off a large piece of foil and put the beets on it, then seal the foil over to form a flat parcel. Put the parcel on a baking tray and bake in the oven until the beets give slightly when you squeeze the parcel; they will take at least 30 minutes, but the cooking time will depend on their size. Test that they are cooked by unwrapping the parcel and sticking a knife in one—it should go in gently, and the skin should also be a little wrinkled.

Carefully unwrap the parcel and allow the beets to cool until they can just be handled. Then slide off the skins; these should come away easily, but may need encouragement with a knife. Put the peeled beets to one side. (If using cooked beets, see tip below; clean them if necessary and pop them in a preheated oven for 5 minutes to warm up—they just need to be warm, not recooked.)

Divide the salad leaves between two plates. Chop the warm beets and scatter the pieces over the leaves. Then rinse the feta cheese, pat dry on paper towels, and crumble it evenly over the beets. Scatter the red onion on top, to taste. Make a dressing by whisking together the olive oil, lemon juice, and thyme leaves in a small bowl and pour it over the salad. Add some black pepper and serve immediately.

Tip:

▶ If it is impossible to find raw beets, use cooked ones—just omit the roasting instructions; instead, warm briefly as instructed in the method above. If the only raw beets you can find are enormous, then definitely use smaller cooked ones. The only beets to avoid are those pickled in vinegar!

Tuna and white bean salad
Serves 2

15 oz (1 x 400 g) can of
   white beans or chickpeas
1 garlic clove, peeled but
   whole
1 tbsp olive oil
1 tsp balsamic vinegar
½ tsp Dijon mustard
squeeze of lemon juice
10 scallions, finely sliced
5 radishes, trimmed, halved,
   and finely sliced
small handful of flat-leaf
   parsley (optional), finely
   chopped

SERVINGS		NUTRITIONAL INFO	
Carbohydrate	0	Calories	281
Protein	4	Carbohydrate	25 g
Fat	1	Protein	26 g
Dairy	0	Fiber	11 g
Fruit	0	Salt	0.4 g
Vegetables	1½		

5½–6½ oz (1 x 160–185 g)
   canned solid white
   albacore tuna in spring
   water
black pepper
1 bag arugula or similarly
   strong-tasting salad
   leaves, about 5 oz (140 g)

Drain and rinse the beans and put them in a pot with the garlic. Cover with fresh water, put the pot over medium to high heat, and bring the beans to a simmer. Turn the heat off and cover the pot; set aside for a couple of minutes while making the dressing.

   Put the olive oil, vinegar, and mustard in a small bowl and squeeze in some lemon juice. Then whisk well to combine all the ingredients into a vinaigrette dressing. Drain the warm beans, remove the garlic clove, and put the beans in a large bowl. Pour the dressing over them and stir well. Set aside for 10 minutes or so to cool down.

   Add the sliced scallions and radishes to the beans, then the parsley (if using), and stir everything together.

Drain the tuna and flake the fish onto the beans, keeping the flakes as large as possible. Add some black pepper and then carefully mix the tuna and the beans together, trying not to break up the tuna too much. Divide the salad leaves between two plates and spoon the tuna and bean salad on top. Serve immediately.

Tip:

▶ You can use any canned bean, or a mixture, in this salad, except green beans!

Tabbouleh

Serves 4

3½ oz (100 g) couscous or
bulgur wheat
juice of 1 large lemon
2 large bunches of flat-leaf
parsley, about 7 oz
(200 g)
small bunch of fresh mint
3 large tomatoes, finely
chopped
2 medium red onions, finely
chopped

1 tbsp olive oil
black pepper

SERVINGS		NUTRITIONAL INFO	
Carbohydrate	1	Calories	140
Protein	0	Carbohydrate	24 g
Fat	½	Protein	5 g
Dairy	0	Fiber	5 g
Fruit	0	Salt	<0.1 g
Vegetables	2		

Put the couscous or bulgur wheat in a bowl and cover it well with boiling water (or follow the instructions on the package). Stir well, then cover the bowl and set it to one side for about 5 minutes; then stir it again, breaking up any lumps. Test a few grains—they should be soft—but leave for another few minutes if they are not. Drain off any excess water in a strainer and squeeze the grains dry by pressing with the back of a wooden spoon. Rinse out the empty bowl and dry it off, then pour in the lemon juice. Put the warm grains back in the bowl and stir it well to incorporate the lemon juice.

Discard the tough stalks of the parsley and mint (cut these off while the herbs are still in bunches). Finely chop the leaves and put in a large bowl, then add the chopped tomatoes and onion. Add the couscous or bulgur wheat and the olive oil and some black pepper. Combine everything together thoroughly, check the seasoning, and serve.

Tips:

▶ This refreshing Mediterranean salad should be made with lots of parsley, and it's delicious as an accompaniment to cold chicken, such as "Baked chicken with rosemary" (see page 275).

▶ If available, choose whole wheat couscous over ordinary couscous; just follow the instructions on the package.

Red cabbage coleslaw with nuts and seeds
Serves 2

3½ oz (100 g) red cabbage
2 medium carrots, peeled
1 large celery stick (optional)
1 medium red onion
3 tbsp low-fat mayonnaise
4 walnut halves, chopped
2 tsp pumpkin seeds
black pepper

SERVINGS		NUTRITIONAL INFO	
Carbohydrate	0	Calories	194
Protein	0	Carbohydrate	15 g
Fat	2	Protein	4 g
Dairy	0	Fiber	6 g
Fruit	0	Salt	0.7 g
Vegetables	2½		

Using a large knife, finely shred the cabbage and put it in a large mixing bowl. Grate the carrots using a coarse grater and put them in the bowl too. Pull the strings off the outside of the celery, slice it lengthwise, and then finely chop. Next, slice the onion into rings and cut these into sections. Add the chopped celery and onions to the bowl and give everything a good stir, mixing it well.

Add the mayonnaise and a good grind of black pepper to the bowl and then stir again to mix the mayonnaise with all the vegetables. If you are serving the coleslaw immediately, chop the walnuts and scatter these over the coleslaw with the pumpkin seeds. If you plan to serve the salad later, cover the coleslaw and refrigerate it, then add the nuts and seeds just before serving.

Tips:

▶ This healthy coleslaw is good by itself, or perhaps with a whole wheat crusty roll or whole grain crackers. It's also delicious with cold chicken and makes a great packed lunch.

▶ When red cabbage isn't available, just use white cabbage.

Fish and seafood

Shrimp with beans, tomatoes, and thyme
Serves 2

15 oz (1 x 400 g) can kidney
beans
8 (250 g) fresh tomatoes
7 oz (200 g) raw shrimp
2 tsp olive oil
1 garlic clove, finely chopped
1 sprig thyme
black pepper

SERVINGS		NUTRITIONAL INFO	
Carbohydrate	0	Calories	241
Protein	4	Carbohydrate	25 g
Fat	½	Protein	27 g
Dairy	0	Fiber	9 g
Fruit	0	Salt	0.6 g
Vegetables	1½		

Drain and rinse the beans. Chop the tomatoes roughly and rinse the shrimp under cold water.

Put the olive oil in a nonstick frying pan over medium heat. When it is warm, add the tomatoes and the garlic and cook them together for a couple of minutes. Strip the leaves off the thyme and add them to the pan, then add the beans. Add the shrimp and cook for about 5 minutes, until they turn pink and are cooked through. During this time add a little water to keep the mixture from sticking to the bottom of the pan; a couple of tablespoons should be enough—the dish should be lightly sauced—but this will depend on how juicy the tomatoes were. Check for seasoning and add black pepper to taste. Serve immediately, perhaps with whole wheat or crusty multi-grain bread to mop up the sauce.

Tip:
▶ If you cannot buy raw shrimp, you can use cooked shrimp instead, but this will increase the salt content. Cooked shrimp

should only be gently warmed to avoid overcooking. Add after you have cooked the beans for about 5 minutes.

Quick fish curry

Serves 4

1 lb 9 oz (750 g) thick cod fillet

2 tsp canola or other neutral-tasting oil

2 medium onions, finely chopped

2 garlic cloves, finely chopped

2 tsp garam masala

½ tsp cayenne pepper

½ tsp turmeric

black pepper

1 tbsp tomato purée

1½ cups (12 fl oz) water

squeeze of lemon juice

To serve:

1 cup (8 oz) basmati rice, brown if possible

SERVINGS		NUTRITIONAL INFO	
With rice			
Carbohydrate	2	Calories	415
Protein	3	Carbohydrate	56 g
Fat	0	Protein	40 g
Dairy	0	Fiber	4 g
Fruit	0	Salt	0.3 g
Vegetables	½		

The rice will probably take longer than the curry (depending on the brand and whether it is brown or white), so prepare it according to the instructions on the package before starting the curry itself.

Carefully remove the skin from the fish and discard any bones you come across, then cut the fish into pieces no smaller than about 1 in square. Heat the oil in a pan or heatproof casserole over medium heat and add the onion and garlic. Cook these for about 5 minutes, or until the onion begins to soften but has not begun to take on much color.

Add the garam masala, cayenne pepper, turmeric, and some black pepper and stir, then add the tomato purée. Stir once, then quickly add the water and let the sauce come to a steady but gentle simmer. Carefully add the pieces of fish and cover the pan.

Cook the curry for 10 minutes, then lift the lid and check that the fish is cooking well. If the sauce is nicely reduced, put the lid back on and cook the curry for another 5 minutes; if there is still plenty of sauce, leave the lid off to reduce it further, but be careful the curry doesn't stick to the bottom of the pan. It is important not to stir the curry too much or the pieces of fish will break up. Just before serving, add a squeeze of lemon juice and a little pepper (taste before seasoning) and stir carefully; serve the curry with the rice.

Tip:

▶ This delicious fish curry could be served with steamed spinach.

Kedgeree with fresh salmon

Serves 2

2 small salmon fillets, skin removed, about 3½ oz (100 g) each
1 large egg
¼ cup (2 oz) basmati rice, preferably brown
1 tsp canola oil
1 medium onion, peeled and chopped

SERVINGS		NUTRITIONAL INFO	
Using brown basmati rice			
Carbohydrate	1	Calories	388
Protein	4	Carbohydrate	31 g
Fat	0	Protein	28 g
Dairy	0	Fiber	3 g
Fruit	0	Salt	0.3 g
Vegetables	½		

1 garlic clove, finely chopped   handful of flat-leaf parsley,
   (optional)   chopped
½ tsp garam masala or mild
   curry powder

Put the salmon in a microwaveable dish. Cover it with plastic wrap, puncture the film in several places, and microwave at full power for 1½ minutes. Check to see that the fish flakes easily and set it aside if it does so (if not, give it another 30 seconds, continuing until it is ready). If you haven't got a microwave, put the salmon fillets in a pan and add enough water to come halfway up the sides. Poach over medium heat until the fish flakes easily, which will probably take less than 10 minutes, depending on the thickness of the fillets. Flake the fish and set it to one side. Hard-boil the egg, rinse under cold water, and leave it in cold water to cool down.

Rinse the rice under running water and put it in a nonstick pot. Add ½ cup water and bring to a boil. Lower the heat until the rice is simmering, then cover the pot and cook the rice until most of the water has been absorbed and the rice is tender (check that it isn't sticking). This will take 15–45 minutes depending on whether you use white or brown rice.

While the rice is cooking, peel the hard-boiled egg and cut it into quarters. Heat the oil in a large nonstick frying pan. Cook the chopped onion very gently until it has softened, then add the garlic (if using) and garam masala. Stir to combine.

Add the rice to the pan and stir it well to blend everything together. Then carefully add the flaked fish and stir it, very gently this time, until thoroughly mixed. Make sure the salmon is warmed through, then divide the kedgeree between the serving dishes. Garnish each serving with pieces of hard-boiled egg and a sprinkling of chopped parsley and serve immediately.

Tip:

▶ Kedgeree is often used as a brunch dish, but it makes a great choice for supper too. For supper, serve it with steamed vegetables or a couple of salads—a plain green salad and one featuring tomatoes and scallions would be especially good.

Salmon with lentils
Serves 2

3½ oz (100 g) Puy lentils (uncooked weight)
1 small onion, peeled and halved
1 garlic clove, peeled but whole
1 bay leaf
1 sprig of thyme
½ tsp olive oil
1 tbsp low-fat cream cheese
black pepper

2 salmon fillets, skin removed, approximately 4 oz (120 g) each

SERVINGS		NUTRITIONAL INFO	
Carbohydrate	0	Calories	404
Protein	6	Carbohydrate	28 g
Fat	0	Protein	39 g
Dairy	½	Fiber	7 g
Fruit	0	Salt	0.3 g
Vegetables	½		

Rinse the lentils, then put them in a pot with half of the onion, the garlic clove, bay leaf, and sprig of thyme. Cover with water and bring to a boil. Reduce the heat to a simmer and cook until the lentils are tender but not soft or mushy. This shouldn't take longer than 30 minutes. Drain the lentils and discard the half onion, garlic, bay leaf, and the stalk of the thyme—most of the leaves will have come off.

Finely chop the remaining half onion. Put the oil in a pan over medium heat and fry the onions gently for 3–4 minutes. Add the lentils and heat through, then take off the heat and allow to cool for two or three minutes before stirring in the cream cheese. Season with black pepper and cover the pan to keep the lentils warm while you cook the salmon.

Heat a nonstick frying pan over a medium to high heat. Place the salmon fillets in the pan and cook them gently on one side for about 2 minutes, until they just begin to color. Then turn them over and cook the other side, also for about 2 minutes. Check that the salmon is cooked right through (this will depend on the thickness of the fillets) and take the pan off the heat.

Divide the lentils between two warmed plates. Gently place a fillet of salmon on top of each and serve immediately.

Tip:

▶ Puy lentils are readily available and don't need preliminary soaking. They also have a lovely nutty taste and are really nutritious.

Fish couscous
Serves 4

1 lb (500 g) firm white fish
    (cod or monkfish tail)
14 oz (1 x 400 g) can
    chickpeas
2 tsp olive oil
2 medium onions, finely
    chopped

SERVINGS		NUTRITIONAL INFO	
Carbohydrate	2	Calories	359
Protein	3	Carbohydrate	48 g
Fat	0	Protein	33 g
Dairy	0	Fiber	9 g
Fruit	0	Salt	0.3 g
Vegetables	2		

2 garlic cloves, chopped
1 tsp ground cumin
½ tsp cayenne pepper
½ tsp ras el hanout (or
"Moroccan spice blend"),
optional
2 medium carrots, peeled
and chopped

1 medium red bell pepper,
deseeded and chopped
1 medium yellow bell pepper,
deseeded and chopped
4 tsp tomato purée dissolved
in 1¾ cups (14 fl oz) hot
water
6 oz (175 g) couscous

Cut the fish into large pieces, put them in a bowl, cover, and put in the refrigerator. If you are using monkfish, you may need to fillet it first. Slice the fillets away from the central bone with a really sharp knife, then cut away the membrane on the outside. Discard the bone and membrane and chop the flesh. Drain and rinse the chickpeas thoroughly.

Put the oil in a large pan over medium heat. Add the onions and cook them, stirring, for 5 minutes. Then add the garlic, stir in the spices, and cook for 1 minute more, still stirring well. Add the carrot and peppers to the pan, mixing them in, then add the tomato purée diluted in water. Simmer for 15 minutes, then add the chickpeas and the fish. Add enough water, if necessary, to cover everything—this fish stew should be quite liquid. Partly cover the pan and cook for another 6–10 minutes, depending on the type of fish used. The vegetables and the fish should be cooked but not breaking up, the chickpeas should be soft, and the liquid will have reduced a little.

Toward the end of cooking, prepare the couscous. Either follow the instructions on the package or put the dried couscous in a large bowl and add boiling water to cover it well. Stir with a fork, cover the bowl, and wait until the grains have absorbed most of the water, which will only take a few minutes. Stir a couple of times, then drain the couscous well through a fine strainer.

Put a serving of couscous on each plate and ladle the fish, vegetables, and sauce over it. Serve immediately.

Tip:

▶ If available, choose whole wheat couscous. This recipe also works well with bulgur wheat.

Smoked fish cakes

Serves 4 (makes 8 fish cakes)

1 lb 4 oz (600 g) smoked haddock or trout fillets, skin removed, undyed if possible
14 oz (400 g) new potatoes in their skins, chopped
black pepper
8 scallions, trimmed and finely chopped
1 egg, beaten
1 tbsp whole wheat flour

2 tbsp whole wheat breadcrumbs
2 tbsp canola or other neutral-tasting oil
1 lemon, quartered

SERVINGS		NUTRITIONAL INFO	
Carbohydrate	1½	Calories	319
Protein	2½	Carbohydrate	30 g
Fat	1	Protein	35 g
Dairy	0	Fiber	3 g
Fruit	0	Salt	3.2 g
Vegetables	0		

Cook the fish, either in a microwave or a pan. To microwave, put the fillets in a microwave-proof dish, add a couple of tablespoons of water, cover with plastic wrap, and pierce the wrap in several places with a knife. Then microwave on full power until the fish is cooked and the flesh flakes easily; this should take about 2–3 minutes. Once the fish is done, lift it out of the dish and put on a plate, but keep the cooking liquid. If cooking the fish on the stove, put the fillets in a large pan over a medium heat, cover with water, and poach until done—again, save the cooking liquid. This takes about 5 minutes, depending on the thickness of the fillet.

Boil the potatoes until soft, then drain. Add some black pepper and a little of the fish cooking liquid—they should be quite dry—and mash them until they are smooth, then transfer to a bowl. Flake the fish well and add it to the potatoes, then add the scallions. Add about two-thirds of the beaten egg and stir everything together with a wooden spoon. Then cover the bowl and put it in the refrigerator for 30 minutes or so.

Cover a large baking sheet (or two smaller ones) with parchment paper or foil. Dust the flour onto a board or work surface and put the rest of the beaten egg in a bowl and the breadcrumbs on a plate. Take the fish cake mixture out of the refrigerator and, using a spoon, divide the mix into eight. One at a time, rub your hands with the flour and roll each serving between your hands into a ball, then press it gently into a fat fish cake shape. Dip each cake briefly in the reserved beaten egg, then roll in the breadcrumbs, covering all the surfaces. Put the finished fish cakes on the baking sheet. When they are all done, put the sheet in the refrigerator for 20–30 minutes to chill.

Put the oil in a large nonstick frying pan over medium heat. Once it is hot, carefully put in the fish cakes and cook them gently, turning them over to do each side—how long this takes will depend on how fat they are, but it shouldn't be more than about 8 minutes. Drain them on paper towels and then serve immediately with the lemon quarters and perhaps with steamed spinach or an arugula and tomato salad on the side.

Caribbean shrimp and rice
Serves 2

1 medium tomato

½ cup (3½ oz) long-grain
    brown rice

1 tsp olive oil

1 small onion, peeled and
    finely chopped

2 garlic cloves, crushed

1 red bell pepper, deseeded
    and chopped

1 chili, deseeded and finely
    chopped, or a pinch of
    cayenne pepper

2 cups (16 fl oz) low-salt
    vegetable stock

½ tsp paprika

10½ oz raw jumbo shrimp

handful of cilantro leaves,
    chopped (optional)

SERVINGS		NUTRITIONAL INFO	
Carbohydrate	1½	Calories	405
Protein	3	Carbohydrate	59 g
Fat	0	Protein	33 g
Dairy	0	Fiber	5 g
Fruit	0	Salt	1.6 g
Vegetables	2		

Chop the tomato and put it to one side. Rinse the rice under cold running water.

Put the oil in a large frying pan with a lid (an ordinary pot will do if necessary) and warm it over medium heat. Add the onion, garlic, bell pepper, and the chili, if using, and fry them gently until they soften and begin to change color. Then add the stock, the chopped tomato, the pinch of cayenne (if using instead of chili), and the paprika. Bring the liquid to a simmer and cover the pan.

Add the rice, then simmer on low heat until it is tender and almost all the liquid has been absorbed—the time will vary, so check regularly, but it will probably be about 45 minutes. If the rice shows signs of drying out completely, add a little boiling water; if there seems to be a lot of liquid, increase the temperature slightly to cook it off. As soon as the rice is ready, add the shrimp and cook until pink and cooked through. Take the pan off the heat and serve immediately, with the cilantro leaves scattered on top.

Tips:

▶ Make this dish as hot as you like—just add more chili.

▶ Sliced avocado and a celery salad would make excellent accompaniments.

▶ If you cannot buy raw shrimp, you can use cooked shrimp instead, but they are higher in salt. Cooked shrimp should only be gently warmed to avoid overcooking.

Chicken

Baked chicken with rosemary
Serves 2

2 skinless chicken breasts, about 4 oz (125 g) each
1 tsp olive oil
3 sprigs of rosemary
2 garlic cloves, cut into quarters
juice of 1 lemon

SERVINGS		NUTRITIONAL INFO	
Carbohydrate	0	Calories	159
Protein	4	Carbohydrate	1 g
Fat	0	Protein	28 g
Dairy	0	Fiber	<1 g
Fruit	0	Salt	0.3 g
Vegetables	0		

Preheat the oven to 400°F. Remove the skin from the chicken breasts (if not skinless) and discard it.

Drizzle the oil into an ovenproof dish, swirl it around, and put the dish in the oven until the oil is hot. Take the dish out of the oven and turn the chicken breasts in the oil to seal them and brown them slightly, then take them out and put them on a plate.

Put the whole sprigs of rosemary in the dish, then scatter in the pieces of garlic. Put the chicken breasts on top of the rosemary, right side up. Dilute the lemon juice up to 3½ fl oz (100 ml) with water and pour it over the chicken.

Return the dish to the oven and cook the chicken for 20 minutes. Then turn the breasts over and cook for another 5–10 minutes before turning them the right way up again and cooking until they are done: the juice should run clear when you stick a knife into the thickest part. This will probably take another 10 minutes, depending on the size of the chicken breasts. Once the chicken is ready, lift it out of the dish and allow any excess lemony liquid to run off before serving. Serve the breasts immediately, or chill them thoroughly once they have cooled down.

Tips:

▶ These chicken breasts are ideal hot or cold with steamed vegetables, a tomato salad, or a baked potato.

▶ Pasta makes a good accompaniment when the chicken breasts are hot, especially if you spoon some of the lemony liquid over the pasta before serving.

▶ Cold and sliced, these chicken breasts are great as a sandwich ingredient or as part of a salad.

Mediterranean chicken casserole
Serves 4

3 medium onions, peeled

1 tbsp olive oil

4 chicken breasts, skin removed, about 4 oz (125 g) each

1 large green bell pepper, deseeded and chopped

2 garlic cloves, peeled and finely chopped

14 oz (1 x 400 g) can chopped tomatoes

2 sprigs of thyme, leaves stripped

SERVINGS		NUTRITIONAL INFO	
Carbohydrate	0	Calories	233
Protein	4	Carbohydrate	14 g
Fat	1	Protein	31 g
Dairy	0	Fiber	4 g
Fruit	0	Salt	0.9 g
Vegetables	1½		

1 sprig of fresh oregano or marjoram (if available), leaves stripped

½ cup (4 fl oz) chicken or vegetable stock

15 black olives, pitted and halved

Slice one of the onions into rings and finely chop the other two. Heat the olive oil in a large pan or heatproof casserole over medium to high heat. Cut the chicken breasts into pieces no larger than ½ in square, and add them to the pan once the oil is hot. You may need to do this in several batches to prevent overcrowding. Stir the pieces around, sealing and browning them slightly, and then lift them out of the pan and put aside.

Lower the heat and add the onions, bell pepper, and garlic. Cook gently in what remains of the oil until they are beginning to soften and brown, stirring so they do not stick to the bottom of the pan. Then return the chicken pieces to the pan and add the chopped tomatoes. Add the stripped leaves from the thyme and oregano or marjoram. Finally, add the stock, bring to a simmer, then cover the pan and cook gently for about 30–35 minutes. Check it and give it a stir halfway through the cooking time.

After 35 minutes, add the olives and check the level of liquid. The final sauce should be thick, so if it looks a little thin, raise the heat and take off the lid. Cook for another 10 minutes, or until the chicken is really tender and the vegetables are soft and melting. Check for seasoning, stir gently, and serve.

Tips:

▶ This chicken dish is lovely by itself with steamed vegetables or a green salad, but it is also good with boiled rice or new potatoes.

▶ A pinch of dried mixed herbs—herbes de Provence or an Italian blend—can be used instead of the fresh thyme and marjoram.

▶ This recipe freezes very well.

Chicken tagine with carrots and chickpeas
Serves 4

1 lb (425 g) chicken breasts, skin removed

2 tsp olive oil

1 medium onion, roughly chopped

3 medium carrots, chopped

¼ tsp ground ginger

¼ tsp cinnamon

SERVINGS		NUTRITIONAL INFO	
Carbohydrate	½	Calories	217
Protein	4	Carbohydrate	16 g
Fat	0	Protein	27 g
Dairy	0	Fiber	5 g
Fruit	0	Salt	0.3 g
Vegetables	1		

juice of half a lemon   *2 tsp tomato purée*

7½ oz (1 x 210 g) can   *about 2 cups (16 fl oz) water*

  chickpeas, drained and   *or chicken stock*

  rinsed   *2 tsp honey*

Cut the chicken breasts into pieces no bigger than ½ in square. Heat the oil in a large, heavy-bottomed saucepan or heatproof casserole over medium heat. Add the chopped onion and carrots and cook gently until the onion just begins to change color.

Add the chicken pieces and stir for a minute or so. Keep stirring to make sure the chicken pieces don't stick to the bottom of the pan and then add the spices and the lemon juice. Stir everything well to coat the chicken in the spices, then add the chickpeas, tomato purée, and enough stock or water to cover the chicken.

Cook for 30 minutes, uncovered, then add the honey. Continue cooking for another 10 minutes, or until the sauce is much reduced. If you're intending to serve the tagine with couscous or bulgur wheat, don't reduce the sauce too much.

Tip:
▶ Instead of the carrots, substitute half a small butternut squash, peeled, deseeded, and chopped.

Chicken fajitas
Serves 4

1 lb (500 g) skinless chicken   *½ tsp paprika*

  breasts   *1 tsp ground cumin*

2 limes

1 red chili, deseeded and
   finely chopped, or ½ tsp
   chili powder
black pepper
2 tsp olive oil
1 red bell pepper, deseeded
   and finely chopped
1 green bell pepper, deseeded
   and finely chopped
1 medium red onion
1 tsp tomato purée

SERVINGS		NUTRITIONAL INFO	
Carbohydrate	2	Calories	381
Protein	4	Carbohydrate	49 g
Fat	0	Protein	36 g
Dairy	½	Fiber	5 g
Fruit	0	Salt	0.8 g
Vegetables	2		

To serve:
salad leaves
bunch of cilantro, leaves only
5 oz low-fat plain yogurt
4 tortilla wraps

Cut the chicken breast into fine strips, no longer than 1½ in and no larger than ¼ in deep and wide. Squeeze one of the limes into a large mixing bowl and add the paprika, cumin, chili or chili powder, and a good grinding of black pepper. Add a teaspoon of olive oil as well, then stir everything together. Add the chicken and mix it in with a wooden spoon. Set the bowl to one side.

In the meantime, prepare the peppers and cut the onion in half and then into slices. Add the vegetables to the chicken bowl, together with the juice of the other lime, and stir well.

Put some crisp salad leaves on each serving plate, and remove the leaves from the cilantro. Pour the yogurt into a small bowl. If you want to heat the tortillas in the oven, preheat it and put them in (following the instructions on the package) or use a microwave.

Warm a large nonstick frying pan or wok on high heat and add a teaspoon of oil. When smoking, add the chicken mixture.

Cook, stirring constantly to prevent it from burning, for 5 minutes. Then add the tomato purée and stir it in. Continue cooking and stirring for 1 minute, or until you are sure the chicken is cooked—it should be beginning to crisp a little at the edges and will be opaque all the way through. Remove from the heat.

Then assemble the fajitas: spoon some yogurt on each tortilla wrap, scatter some cilantro leaves over it, and divide the chicken among them. Add a little more yogurt and then fold the tortilla over. Serve immediately.

Tip:

▶ You can also use turkey breast or steak in this recipe instead of the chicken and include some guacamole (see page 194) when you fold the fajitas.

Meat

Homemade classic burgers

Serves 4 (makes 4 burgers)

1 lb ground sirloin

black pepper

1 large sprig of thyme, leaves
   stripped

2 tsp Dijon or grainy
   mustard (optional)

2 small egg yolks, or
   1 large one

SERVINGS		NUTRITIONAL INFO	
Carbohydrate	0	Calories	254
Protein	4	Carbohydrate	<1 g
Fat	0	Protein	29 g
Dairy	0	Fiber	0 g
Fruit	0	Salt	0.6 g
Vegetables	0		

Put the beef in a bowl, grind some black pepper over it, and mix it well with a wooden spoon, breaking up any chunks. Then add the leaves from the thyme, the mustard, and the egg yolks and combine. The mixture will come together, but do not overwork the meat as it will toughen the burgers. Divide it into four equal amounts and form into four patties.

Preheat the broiler. Put a large piece of foil on the broiler pan, then carefully lift the patties onto the foil with a spatula. Cook the burgers under the grill for 5–10 minutes, turning once until they are done to your satisfaction. How long this takes will depend on how thick the patties are as well as how you like them done—rare, medium, or well done. Serve immediately.

Vegetarian alternative:

Drain and rinse two 15-oz cans of kidney beans in water. Put them in a pan, cover with fresh water, and bring to a boil; then drain the beans again (this makes them easier to mash) and put them in a bowl. Add

SERVINGS		NUTRITIONAL INFO	
Carbohydrate	1	Calories	248
Protein	2	Carbohydrate	41 g
Fat	0	Protein	15 g
Dairy	0	Fiber	10 g
Fruit	0	Salt	0.8 g
Vegetables	0		

1 cup (3½ oz) whole wheat breadcrumbs and mash together with the beans, then add the thyme, mustard, and egg yolks and stir everything thoroughly. Form into 4 patties, as above, then put them on a baking sheet and broil for 5–6 minutes on each side.

Tips:

▶ These burgers are simple, healthy, and quick to make, and you can vary the flavorings to suit your personal taste. Try adding some ground cumin, finely chopped chili, and maybe cilantro leaves for a hot and spicy burger, or add a bit of cinnamon and cumin for a North African tang.

▶ Baked potatoes and a tomato salad would make a great accompaniment.

Marinated lamb and red onion kebabs with a yogurt and herb sauce
Serves 2

8 oz boneless lamb shoulder
3 tbsp low-fat plain yogurt
1 tsp olive oil
1 bay leaf
black pepper
1 medium red onion

SERVINGS		NUTRITIONAL INFO	
Protein	4	Calories	374
Fat	0	Carbohydrate	22 g
Dairy	1½	Protein	36 g
Fruit	0	Fiber	2 g
Vegetables	½	Salt	0.6 g

For the sauce:
8 oz (250 g) low- or no-fat
  Greek yogurt
large handful of mint leaves,
  finely chopped
pinch of paprika

To serve:
handful of cilantro leaves

Note: The lamb needs to marinate for several hours or overnight—if it goes into its marinade and into the refrigerator at the start of the day, it will be ready to cook that night.

Cut the lamb into ½-in cubes and discard any fat that is easily detached. Put the lamb cubes into a bowl and spoon the 3 tablespoons of yogurt and oil over them. Add the bay leaf and turn the meat over in the yogurt until thoroughly coated. Grind a little black pepper on top, cover the bowl with plastic wrap, and put it in the refrigerator to marinate.

If you intend to use bamboo skewers for the kebabs, soak them in water for half an hour before you cook. Make the yogurt and herb sauce by putting the Greek yogurt and chopped mint leaves into a bowl. Stir, then sprinkle a little paprika over the top. Pop the dressing in the refrigerator while you prepare and cook the kebabs.

Preheat the broiler. Cut the red onion into quarters, then separate each quarter into individual pieces and take the meat out of the refrigerator. Thread pieces of onion onto the skewers alternately with cubes of meat, then rest the ends of the completed skewers over a roasting pan or baking sheet so the meat is suspended above it.

Put the kebabs under the broiler and cook, turning them a couple of times until they are done to your taste—this will probably take about 10–15 minutes. Serve immediately with a dollop of the yogurt sauce sprinkled with cilantro leaves.

Thai-style stir-fried beef with lime, red onion, and cucumber

Serves 2

8 oz stir-fry beef or beef
   sirloin
1 lemongrass stick
2 limes
1 red chili (or to taste)
½ cucumber
1 medium red onion

SERVINGS		NUTRITIONAL INFO	
Carbohydrate	2	Calories	447
Protein	4	Carbohydrate	57 g
Fat	½	Protein	34 g
Dairy	0	Fiber	5 g
Fruit	0	Salt	0.2 g
Vegetables	2		

4 scallions

*2 tsp canola or other neutral-
tasting oil*

To serve:

*½ cup (120 g) brown
basmati rice*

Marinate the beef for 30 minutes beforehand: if using beef sirloin, cut it into fine strips first. Slice the lemongrass stick in half lengthwise, flatten the bulbous end, and put it into a bowl with the juice of one of the limes. Add the beef, cover the bowl, and set it aside.

Put the rice on to cook (follow the instructions on the package). Get everything ready for the stir-fry. Cut the chili in half, scrape out the seeds, and chop it very finely.

Peel half of one side of the cucumber and then, using a potato peeler, remove several very fine strips and put them to one side. Cut the rest of the cucumber into fine batons about 1½ in long. Cut the onion in half and then slice it into fine semicircles. Chop the scallions finely and put some of the white parts with the thin cucumber strips.

Heat the oil in a wok or large nonstick frying pan over high heat. Take the beef out of the bowl and shake off the lemon-grass. Once the oil is almost smoking, add the beef to the wok. Stir-fry, stirring constantly, for about 3 minutes, until the beef is cooked on all sides. Lift it out of the wok and set aside on a plate, then pour any lime juice from the marinade into the hot wok with the juice of the second lime—it will sizzle. Add the red onion, chili, the cucumber batons, and the bulk of the scal-lions. Stir-fry for 2–3 minutes, until they have taken on color and softened. Then return the beef and any juices to the wok and stir-fry for another minute.

Drain the rice and divide it between two plates. Put the beef stir-fry on top, then garnish with the raw cucumber strips and scallion slices. Squeeze one of the lime skins to get a few extra drops of lime over each plate and serve immediately.

Beef meatballs with sauce
Serves 4

14 oz ground sirloin

2 medium onions

4 garlic cloves

large sprig thyme, leaves
    stripped, or 1 tsp dried
    mixed Italian herbs

black pepper

4 tsp olive oil

3 cups (7 oz) mushrooms,
    sliced

15-oz (1 x 400 g) can
    chopped tomatoes, or a
    double quantity of
    "Universal tomato sauce"
    (see page 290)

About 1 cup (8 fl oz) water

SERVINGS		NUTRITIONAL INFO	
Carbohydrate	0	Calories	256
Protein	3	Carbohydrate	10 g
Fat	½	Protein	25 g
Dairy	0	Fiber	3 g
Fruit	0	Salt	0.3 g
Vegetables	1½		

Put the ground sirloin in a bowl. Finely chop one of the onions and two of the garlic cloves and add them to the meat. Scatter the herbs over the meat and add a good grinding of black pepper, then stir everything together well with a wooden spoon. Form the mixture into 24 small balls, each about half the size of a golf ball.

Heat two teaspoons of oil in a frying pan. Carefully transfer the meatballs to the pan and brown them on all sides (this can be done in batches). Remove them from the pan and put them on a plate. Wipe the pan with a piece of paper towel and add the rest of the oil. Chop the remaining onion and garlic cloves, and fry them gently until they just begin to color. Add the mushrooms and cook for a couple of minutes—they should just begin to brown.

Pour the tomatoes or "Universal tomato sauce" into a measuring cup and add enough water or vegetable stock to make 2½ cups of liquid. Transfer the onion mixture to a large saucepan, and add the tomato sauce. Carefully place the meatballs in the pan and bring the sauce to a boil, then reduce the heat to a gentle simmer, cover the pan, and cook for 30 minutes. Check during this time at 10-minute intervals to ensure that the sauce isn't sticking to the bottom of the pan and lower the heat if necessary. If the sauce seems very liquid, increase the heat a little for the final 10 minutes and take the lid off.

Tip:

▶ These meatballs are delicious with pasta or some boiled rice.

Vegetarian

Crunchy stuffed peppers with arugula and raita

Serves 2

¼ cup long-grain brown rice
3 large red bell peppers (or
  one red, one yellow, and
  one orange)
1½ tsp olive oil
1 large onion, chopped
2 garlic cloves, finely chopped

SERVINGS		NUTRITIONAL INFO	
Carbohydrate	1½	Calories	431
Protein	0	Carbohydrate	63 g
Fat	2	Protein	15 g
Dairy	½	Fiber	12 g
Fruit	0	Salt	0.2 g
Vegetables	5		

4⅓ oz mushrooms, trimmed
   and sliced
3 tsp pine nuts
10 almonds, roughly
   chopped
black pepper
about ½ cup water

For the salad:
1 bag arugula
1 tsp lemon juice

For the raita:
3½ oz plain low-fat yogurt
2-in piece of cucumber, peeled

Cook the rice according to the package instructions.

Preheat the oven to 375°F. Cut the peppers in half through the stalks and deseed them without removing the stalk (leaving the stalks on helps the peppers to hold the stuffing). Keeping the peppers intact while removing the seeds is a bit tricky, but using scissors makes it easier.

Put half a teaspoon of oil on a piece of paper towel and wipe the outside of the peppers, then put them on a rimmed baking sheet, open side up. Bake for 12–15 minutes, depending on their size.

Heat the remaining teaspoon of oil in a nonstick frying pan and add the onion. Cook it for 5 minutes and then add the garlic and the mushrooms. Continue cooking for about 4 minutes, or until the mushrooms and onions are beginning to color, then add the pine nuts, almonds, and a good grinding of black pepper. Stir everything together and take the pan off the heat. Drain the cooked rice and mix it in with the mushrooms and nuts.

Carefully lift the pepper shells off the baking sheet and transfer them to an ovenproof dish (ceramic or glass). Spoon the stuffing into the shells and then pour the water around them—there should be enough to just cover the base of the dish. Put the dish into the oven and bake for 20 minutes.

Prepare the salad and yogurt sauce while the peppers are cooking. Put the arugula leaves in a serving bowl and toss them together with the lemon juice. Spoon the yogurt into a small bowl. Grate the cucumber into a sieve; squeeze out as much liquid as possible and then stir the cucumber into the yogurt. When the peppers are ready, carefully lift them out of whatever water remains in the dish with a large slotted spoon and put them on serving plates. Add a generous spoonful of the yogurt sauce and serve, accompanied by the lemony arugula. A tomato salsa is another refreshing accompaniment.

Pasta arrabbiata (and universal tomato sauce)
Serves 2

1 red chili, or to taste
½ tsp olive oil
1 small onion, chopped
2 garlic cloves, finely chopped
1 8-oz (1 x 227 g) can
  chopped tomatoes
5 oz dried whole wheat penne
basil leaves

SERVINGS		NUTRITIONAL INFO	
For Pasta arrabbiata			
Carbohydrate	2	Calories	196
Protein	0	Carbohydrate	45 g
Fat	0	Protein	10 g
Dairy	0	Fiber	9 g
Fruit	0	Salt	0.3 g
Vegetables	1½		
For sauce only			
Carbohydrate	0	Calories	48
Protein	0	Carbohydrate	7 g
Fat	0	Protein	2 g
Dairy	0	Fiber	2 g
Fruit	0	Salt	0.1 g
Vegetables	1½		

Be careful when preparing chilies—cut off the top, slice the chili in half lengthwise, and scrape out the seeds. Then chop the chili finely and put it to one side.

To make the tomato sauce, heat the oil in a small pot and add the onion, garlic, and chili. Stir them together and cook very gently for about 10 minutes, or until the onion is transparent and soft. Raise the heat and add the canned tomatoes. Simmer the sauce until it is reduced by half.

While the sauce is simmering, cook the pasta. Put a large pot of water on to boil. Cook the pasta until it is just ready—about 10 minutes.

You can serve the tomato sauce either as it is or as a smooth sauce. If you want a smooth sauce, put a small strainer over a bowl and pour the sauce into the strainer. Push it through the strainer with a wooden spoon and scrape the thick sauce into the bowl from the underside of the strainer. Discard the pulp, return the sauce to a clean pot, and warm it through.

When the pasta is ready, drain it and put it back in the pot. Add the sauce, either chunky or smooth, and stir thoroughly to combine. Divide the sauced pasta into two, scatter with a few torn basil leaves, and serve.

Universal tomato sauce

For an all-purpose tomato sauce, make the sauce in the same way as described here, but leave out the chili and include some herbs if you wish—thyme, basil, and oregano are particularly good. The sauce should generally be smooth, but that depends on how you wish to use it. It is easy to increase the quantities to make more, and any extra sauce can be kept in the refrigerator for two days. It also freezes beautifully.

Tip:

▶ This pasta dish should be spicy hot, but not so hot that it's impossible to eat—and it's lightly sauced.

▶ The basic tomato sauce, without the chili, can be used in many other recipes.

▶ Serve the pasta with cooked shrimp or a sliced roast chicken breast on top.

Boston baked beans
Serves 5

2 14-oz (2 x 400 g) cans
    cannellini beans
1 tsp olive oil
1 small carrot, finely chopped
1 medium onion, finely
    chopped
1 celery stick, finely chopped
2 garlic cloves, chopped
¼ tsp cayenne pepper
1 tsp dried oregano, or a good
    handful of fresh oregano
2 tsp clear honey

SERVINGS		NUTRITIONAL INFO	
Carbohydrate	0	Calories	140
Protein	1½	Carbohydrate	25 g
Fat	0	Protein	8 g
Dairy	0	Fiber	8 g
Fruit	0	Salt	0.1 g
Vegetables	1		

1 14-oz (1 x 400 g) can
    chopped tomatoes or
    double quantity of rough
    "Universal tomato sauce"
    (see page 290)

These beans don't have to be baked in the oven; they can be cooked on the stove, as below. If it's more convenient to cook them in the oven, then preheat it to 350°F. Just remember to check on them as they cook.

Drain and rinse the beans and put them to one side. Heat the oil in a nonstick pan and add the chopped carrot, onion, and celery. Cook them gently for 10 minutes, then add the garlic and cook for another 5 minutes.

Stir in the cayenne, then add the beans and stir to combine. Add the oregano, honey, and tomatoes and cook over medium to high heat for 20–30 minutes, stirring regularly, until much of the liquid has evaporated. When the beans are ready, check for seasoning and serve (if you are intending to freeze the beans, don't add seasoning).

Tips:

▶ Homemade baked beans are so much healthier than bought ones, as they contain less salt and sugar.

▶ They freeze really well, making an ideal frozen meal.

Alternative:

Soybeans have a different taste and are very useful for vegetarians, as they provide a complete protein. However, they take longer to cook (you can't use the fresh ones here). Soak 1 cup of dried soybeans overnight, then rinse, cover with lots of water, and boil covered for an hour. Lower the heat and simmer them for another hour. Drain well and use as above.

Orzotto with peas and broad beans
Serves 2

1 tsp olive oil	2¾ oz pearl barley
1 small onion, chopped	2–3 cups hot low-salt
1 garlic clove, finely chopped	vegetable stock
or crushed	3½ oz frozen broad beans

3½ oz frozen peas

black pepper

SERVINGS		NUTRITIONAL INFO	
Carbohydrate	2	Calories	259
Protein	0	Carbohydrate	48 g
Fat	0	Protein	11 g
Dairy	0	Fiber	12 g
Fruit	0	Salt	0.9 g
Vegetables	1½		

Heat the oil in a nonstick pot over medium heat and add the chopped onion and garlic. Cook the onion and garlic gently until transparent, about 10 minutes, and then add the pearl barley. Stir for 2 minutes, coating it in the oil and toasting it in the hot pan, which gives it extra flavor. Then add some of the stock and let it bubble until the stock has been absorbed by the grains. Repeat this until the grains are really beginning to soften, which will take about 35–45 minutes.

When the grains are nearly done, put a pot of water on to boil. Add the broad beans, bring the water back to a boil, and simmer for about 2 minutes. Then add the peas and simmer them until both vegetables are tender. Drain well and as soon as the barley is cooked but still has a bit of bite, add these to the pan and stir them through the orzotto. Check the seasoning, add some black pepper, and serve immediately.

Tips:

▶ A tangy tomato and onion salad makes a good accompaniment to this particular orzotto.

▶ You can substitute all sorts of things instead of peas and broad beans—try mushrooms or butternut squash.

▶ Pearl barley can be very variable in how long it takes to cook; some takes longer and absorbs more liquid before it finally softens, and this can vary with age—the fresher the grains, the less time they take. This is why it's a good idea to cook separately anything you want to put in your orzotto and add it to the barley at the last minute: it won't overcook.

Bean and green pepper chili
Serves 4

2 14-oz (2 x 400 g) cans of kidney beans
1 14-oz (1 x 400 g) can of chopped tomatoes
1 large green bell pepper, deseeded and chopped
1 large onion, finely chopped
2 garlic cloves, crushed
2 tbsp tomato purée
1 tsp cayenne pepper or chili powder (or more, to taste)
1 tsp ground cumin

1 tsp ground coriander
black pepper

To serve:
1 cup basmati rice

SERVINGS		NUTRITIONAL INFO	
Carbohydrate	2	Calories	390
Protein	2	Carbohydrate	80 g
Fat	0	Protein	17 g
Dairy	0	Fiber	14 g
Fruit	0	Salt	0.2 g
Vegetables	2		

Drain and rinse the kidney beans and put them in a large pot over medium heat. Add the tomatoes and then the chopped pepper and onion. Add the crushed garlic, followed by the tomato purée, cayenne or chili powder, cumin, and coriander. Add some black pepper and stir well, then cover. Bring the mixture to a steady simmer and cook for 30 minutes. Cook the rice according to the package instructions.

Check the chili as it cooks and give it a stir. If there seems to be a lot of liquid, take the lid off and increase the temperature;

if it looks a little dry, add a little water. The chili sauce should be thick rather than thin, however. Drain the rice and serve it with the chili.

Tip:

▶ You could substitute Quorn (10½ oz) or TVP (textured vegetable protein) (5 oz) for one of the cans of beans.

Red bell pepper, zucchini, and mushroom lasagne
Serves 4

2 tsp olive oil
1 large onion, chopped
2 garlic cloves, finely
chopped
2 red bell peppers, deseeded
and chopped into ¼-in
dice
1 medium zucchini, sliced
into rings
2 8-oz packages mushrooms,
wiped and chopped
1 14-oz (1 x 400 g) can
chopped tomatoes
1 tsp dried oregano or a
handful of fresh oregano
leaves
8 sheets of lasagne, whole
wheat or spinach
2 tsp grated Parmesan

SERVINGS		NUTRITIONAL INFO	
Carbohydrate	2½	Calories	374
Protein	0	Carbohydrate	50 g
Fat	1	Protein	15 g
Dairy	½	Fiber	10 g
Fruit	0	Salt	0.4 g
Vegetables	3		

For the béchamel sauce:
1¼ oz olive oil margarine
1¼ oz all-purpose flour
1½ cups fat-free milk
pinch of black pepper

Preheat the oven to 350°F. Heat the olive oil in a large saucepan over a medium heat, then add the onion. Cook for 5 minutes or so, until slightly transparent. Add the garlic and stir, then add the peppers. After 5 minutes, add the zucchini, mushrooms, canned tomatoes, and oregano. Cook for another 5–10 minutes, or until the vegetables are softened, then take the pan off the heat and put it to one side.

Put a large pot of water on to boil. Get out a large ovenproof dish about 2½ in deep (ideally, this should be about 9 × 9 in or 11 × 7 in). Then make the sauce. Melt the margarine in a nonstick medium pot over gentle heat. Once it has melted, whisk in the flour and keep whisking until it is completely mixed and starting to change color. Then take the pot off the heat and whisk in the milk very gradually. Put the pot back on the heat and cook the sauce—still whisking—until the sauce thickens, which should only take about 3 minutes. Add a little black pepper, whisk again, and then turn the heat right down or off, in the case of an electric stove. Slip the lasagne sheets into the boiling water two by two, let them soften slightly, then remove and drain on a dish towel, or use them according to the instructions on the package.

Assemble the lasagne. Put a little of the béchamel sauce into the bottom of the ovenproof dish, then spoon about half of the vegetable mixture over it. Top with a layer of half the lasagne sheets. Then pour about half the remaining sauce on top, add another layer of vegetables, and top with the rest of the lasagne. Pour the rest of the sauce over the pasta sheets and sprinkle with the Parmesan. Bake in the oven for 40–45 minutes, until the top is golden and the lasagne is bubbling.

Tip:

▶ If you'd prefer not to use Parmesan, grate some Edam over the top instead.

Zucchini frittata
Serves 2

2 large zucchini (about 5–6 oz total weight), trimmed
2 tsp oil
1 small onion, chopped
4 eggs
black pepper

SERVINGS		NUTRITIONAL INFO	
Carbohydrate	0	Calories	233
Protein	2	Carbohydrate	4 g
Fat	½	Protein	17 g
Dairy	0	Fiber	2 g
Fruit	0	Salt	0.4 g
Vegetables	1½		

Cut the zucchini in half lengthwise and then chop them into slices. Warm 1 teaspoon of the oil in a medium-size ovenproof frying pan, add the zucchini and onion, and cook over gentle heat until soft but not floppy. Set the pan to one side.

Beat the eggs in a bowl with some black pepper. Add the zucchini and onion to the eggs, draining off any liquid first if necessary, and mix everything together well.

Wipe the pan with some paper towels and put it back on the heat. Add the rest of the oil and allow it to heat, then pour in the zucchini-and-egg mixture. Spread it out, pushing the zucchini slices down with a spatula and tilting the pan so the liquid egg runs to the edges. Cook gently, shaking the pan slightly to prevent the frittata from sticking, for about 7 minutes, or until the underside looks brown when you gently lift it up with the spatula.

Heat the broiler and put the pan under it to cook the

top of the frittata. Keep an eye on the frittata, as it will rise and brown quite quickly. Remove the pan from the broiler, slide the frittata onto a plate, and cut it into quarters. Serve immediately.

Tip:

▶ Potato wedges and steamed green beans make delicious accompaniments.

Eggplant curry with chickpeas, rice, and a mango raita

Serves 4

2 medium to large eggplants (about 1 lb 14 oz total weight)

1 14-oz (1 x 400 g) can of chickpeas

½-in-square piece of fresh ginger root, peeled and finely chopped

2 garlic cloves, finely chopped

1 tbsp canola or other neutral-tasting oil

1 large onion, peeled and chopped

1 red chili, finely chopped (optional)

2 tsp garam masala

SERVINGS		NUTRITIONAL INFO	
Carbohydrate	2½	Calories	438
Protein	1	Carbohydrate	81 g
Fat	½	Protein	17 g
Dairy	½	Fiber	14 g
Fruit	0	Salt	0.5 g
Vegetables	3		

6 tbsp tomato purée

about 2 cups boiling water

To serve:

1 cup basmati rice

Mango raita:

10½ oz low-fat plain yogurt

2 tsp mango chutney

Cut the eggplants into slices and then cut the slices into cubes. Drain and rinse the chickpeas and set both to one side. Rinse the rice, put it in a bowl, and cover with cold water. Make the raita by putting the yogurt in a bowl and stirring in the mango chutney. Cover the bowl and put it in the refrigerator.

Chop the ginger and the garlic very finely, going over them with a knife until they are almost minced. Heat the oil in a large pan over medium heat and add the ginger, garlic paste, and chopped onion. Cook, stirring, until the onion is soft but not beginning to color, then add the chili (if using) and the garam masala. Cook for a few seconds, still stirring, and then add the eggplant.

Put the tomato purée in a heatproof bowl and add boiling water; stir, then pour over the eggplant until it is covered. Simmer for 10 minutes. While the eggplant is cooking, put the rice and its soaking water in a pot and cook according to the package instructions.

When the eggplant has been cooking for 10 minutes, add the chickpeas and cover the pan. Continue cooking for another 10 minutes, keeping an eye on the level of sauce and adding a little water if necessary; give it a good stir to prevent it sticking to the bottom of the pan. If there seems to be a lot of sauce, raise the heat for the last few minutes so that some of it can cook off—this should be quite a dry dish. Serve the curry with the rice as soon as both the rice and the eggplant are ready.

Tips:

▶ The yogurt sauce (mango raita) that accompanies this curry can also be made by adding a similar quantity of whatever Indian pickle you like, though mango works particularly well with eggplant.

▶ You can also add grated cucumber or onion to the yogurt for a more authentic raita—squeeze excess moisture out of the cucumber first.

Sweets and Desserts

Lemon and blueberry yogurt cake
Serves 12

1 cup (8 oz) whole wheat flour
2½ tsp baking powder
½ cup (4 oz) superfine sugar
1 cup (8 oz) low-fat Greek yogurt
¼ cup (2 fl oz) canola oil
¾ cup (6 fl oz) 1% milk
juice and zest of 1 lemon

SERVINGS		NUTRITIONAL INFO	
Carbohydrate	1	Calories	174
Protein	½	Carbohydrate	23 g
Fat	½	Protein	6 g
Dairy	0	Fiber	2 g
Fruit	0	Salt	0.1 g
Vegetables	0		

3 eggs, separated
⅔ c (3½ oz) blueberries

Preheat the oven to 350°F.

Lightly grease and line the base of a 7-in springform pan with parchment paper.

Sift the flour, baking powder, and sugar into a large bowl and make a well in the center.

In a separate bowl, beat together the yogurt, canola oil, milk, lemon zest and juice, and the egg yolks. Stir in the blueberries.

In another bowl, whisk the egg whites until stiff but not dry. Pour the yogurt mix into the dry ingredients and fold, using a metal spoon, until just combined. Gently fold in the egg whites until just combined and pour the mixture into the pan. Bake for 30 minutes, until a toothpick inserted into the middle comes out clean. Leave to cool in the pan for 10 minutes before turning out onto a cooling rack.

Yogurt ice cream with raspberries
Serves 6

¾ cup (6 oz) very ripe
  raspberries, fresh or frozen
2 tbsp (1 oz) sugar
2 cups (16 oz) plain low-fat
  yogurt

SERVINGS		NUTRITIONAL INFO	
Carbohydrate	½ ·	Calories	129
Protein	0	Carbohydrate	19 g
Fat	0	Protein	7 g
Dairy	½	Fiber	3 g
Fruit	½	Salt	0.2 g
Vegetables	0		

Check over the raspberries, removing any small pieces of leaf; rinse them briefly and put them in a bowl. If using frozen berries, defrost before proceeding with the rest of the recipe. Add the sugar and stir it into the raspberries, breaking them up; then add the yogurt. Blitz everything together using a handheld blender (or transfer the mixture to a blender).

Give the mixture a final stir to make sure it is smooth and that everything is thoroughly blended together, then pour it into a shallow freezer container or a similar dish you can safely put in the freezer. Freeze the yogurt mixture for an hour, or until crystals form around the edge. Take it out of the freezer and whisk the mixture thoroughly, then return the container to the freezer. Repeat the whisking after another hour (you can use a handheld blender—spoon it into a bowl, blend it, and return it to the freezer container) and then freeze the ice cream for at least another 2 hours, or until solid.

Take the yogurt ice cream out of the freezer about 15 minutes before you want to serve it and leave it at room temperature to soften slightly.

Tips:

▶ You can use any berries with this recipe, as long as they are ripe and juicy.

▶ Yogurt ice cream has a different texture from ice cream made with milk, but whisking it well helps to make it smoother.

Individual lemon and honey cheesecakes
Serves 2

3 tbsp thick rolled oats

2 tsp vegetable oil spread,
  preferably sunflower

pinch ground ginger
  (optional)

½ cup plus 2 tbsp (5 oz)
  plain low-fat cream cheese

1 tbsp low-fat or fat-free
  Greek yogurt

2 tsp clear honey

SERVINGS		NUTRITIONAL INFO	
Carbohydrate	2	Calories	213
Protein	0	Carbohydrate	23 g
Fat	1	Protein	12 g
Dairy	2½	Fiber	2 g
Fruit	0	Salt	0.9 g
Vegetables	0		

zest and juice of half a large
  lemon

Put the oats into a dry pan over medium heat. Stir with a wooden spoon until they suddenly start to smell toasty and change color. Take the pan off the heat, empty the oats into a small bowl, then add the spread and the ground ginger (if using). Mix these together immediately, working the spread in with a wooden spoon; the warmth of the oats will melt it. When thoroughly combined, divide the mixture between two ramekins (or 2 wine or cocktail glasses) and press it into the base. Put the ramekins in the refrigerator for at least an hour.

Take the cream cheese out of the refrigerator 10 minutes before you make the filling so that it is soft enough to work with. Put the cheese, yogurt, and honey in a bowl and beat them together. Add the lemon juice and beat that in too. Carefully divide the mixture between the two ramekins. Level the tops and put them back in the refrigerator for another 3 hours (or more). Just before serving, scatter the top of each cheesecake with the lemon zest.

Crunchy blackberry and apple crumble
Serves 4

2 medium sweet apples
squeeze of lemon juice
Almost 1½ cups (11 oz) ripe
  blackberries

For the crumble topping:
1 c (4 oz) rolled oats
2 tbsp ground almonds
2 tbsp whole wheat flour
1 tbsp light brown sugar

SERVINGS		NUTRITIONAL INFO	
Carbohydrate	1½	Calories	326
Protein	0	Carbohydrate	46 g
Fat	2	Protein	7 g
Dairy	0	Fiber	10 g
Fruit	2	Salt	0.3 g
Vegetables	0		

¼ cup olive oil or similar
  vegetable oil spread
½ tsp cinnamon

Preheat the oven to 350°F. Peel, core, and chop the apples and put them in a bowl. Squeeze some lemon juice over them, then add the blackberries and mix these together well. Put the fruit in a medium-size ovenproof dish (about 7–8 in diameter).

Put the oats, ground almonds, flour, and brown sugar in a bowl and mix them together. Then add the spread and rub it in until the mixture resembles fine breadcrumbs. Add the cinnamon and mix it in too. Spoon the crumble over the fruit and press it down. Put the dish in the oven and bake it for about 30–40 minutes, or until the top is golden brown.

Serve with plain low-fat or fat-free Greek yogurt.

Crêpes

Serves 4 (makes 4 crêpes, using a medium frying pan)

½ c (4 oz) all-purpose flour
1 tbsp whole wheat flour
1 medium egg
1 c (8 fl oz) 1% milk
1 tsp sunflower oil spread per
   crêpe

To serve:
juice of 1 lemon
4 tsp clear honey

SERVINGS		NUTRITIONAL INFO	
Crêpes			
Carbohydrate	1	Calories	166
Protein	0	Carbohydrate	23 g
Fat	1	Protein	7 g
Dairy	0	Fiber	1 g
Fruit	0	Salt	0.2 g
Vegetables	0		
With Honey			
Carbohydrate	1½	Calories	189
Protein	0	Carbohydrate	29 g
Fat	1	Protein	7 g
Dairy	0	Fiber	1 g
Fruit	0	Salt	0.2 g
Vegetables	0		

Put the flours into a bowl and break in the egg. Using a whisk, stir these together, breaking up the yolk, then gradually add the milk, whisking until you have a mixture the consistency of cream without lumps.

Put a nonstick frying pan over high heat. When the pan is hot, add a little spread and let it melt; tip the pan to spread it over the surface. Now add the batter—about 3–4 tablespoons per crêpe, though this will depend on the size of pan: crêpes should be thinner than standard pancakes. Again tip the pan in all directions, letting the batter run to the sides. Put the pan back on the heat and after a couple of minutes' cooking, gently lift one side of the crepe: it should be lightly browned. Flip it over (a spatula or palette knife is useful) and cook the underside—this will take less time; allow 1 minute.

You can either make one crêpe and store the rest of the batter in the refrigerator or you can make the whole batch. If making all four in one go, once the first crêpe is cooked, slide it onto a warm plate, cover lightly with foil, and keep warm in a coolish oven while you continue. Once ready to eat, slide the crêpe onto a serving plate, drizzle with lemon juice and a teaspoon of clear honey, and roll it over. Serve immediately.

Tip:
▶ Instead of honey, serve with chopped banana or mixed berries and a spoonful of low-fat Greek yogurt.

Apricot and apple fruit salad
Serves 2

4 dried apricots, chopped

¼ cup (2 fl oz) apple juice, chilled

4 fresh apricots

2 small sweet apples

SERVINGS		NUTRITIONAL INFO	
Carbohydrate	0	Calories	94
Protein	0	Carbohydrate	23 g
Fat	0	Protein	2 g
Dairy	0	Fiber	5 g
Fruit	2	Salt	<0.1 g
Vegetables	0		

Put the dried apricots in a bowl. Add the apple juice, cover the bowl, and leave it in the refrigerator for at least an hour. Cut up the fresh apricots: halve and remove the pits first, then chop into smaller pieces and add them to the bowl. Cut the apples into fine slices and stir these in. Divide the fruit between two serving bowls and spoon any apple juice that remains in the larger bowl over them. Serve immediately.

Tip:
▶ Fresh apricots are delicious, but very seasonal. If you can't find them, choose ripe plums instead.

Baked nectarines stuffed with nuts
Serves 2

2 ripe nectarines

2 level tbsp ground almonds

1 tsp sugar

15 almonds, chopped

½ cup (4 fl oz) orange juice

1 tsp shelled unsalted pistachios, chopped (optional; if not using, add 5 more almonds)

Preheat the oven to 400°F. You will need a small oven-proof dish just big enough to hold four halves of nectarine so that they don't topple over.

Halve the nectarines, cutting through to the pit. Twist one half of each fruit to release it from the pit and

SERVINGS		NUTRITIONAL INFO	
Carbohydrate	0	Calories	219
Protein	0	Carbohydrate	18 g
Fat	3	Protein	7 g
Dairy	0	Fiber	4 g
Fruit	1½	Salt	<0.1 g
Vegetables	0		

then cut the pit out of the other half. Place the halves in the ovenproof dish, cut side up.

Put the ground almonds into a bowl and add the sugar and chopped nuts, then moisten the mixture with a little orange juice until it holds together. Mix well and then spoon it into the cavities left by the nectarine pits. Pour the rest of the orange juice into the dish around the fruit.

Cover the dish lightly with foil and put it into the oven. Bake for 15 minutes, then remove the foil. Cook for another 5 minutes, or until soft. Gently lift each fruit out of the ovenproof dish with a slotted spoon, and put it in a serving bowl. Spoon a little of the juice around each and serve immediately.

Chocolate and orange mousse
Note: This recipe contains raw eggs and is therefore not suitable to be shared with anyone who is pregnant or in poor health.
Serves 4

4 oz dark chocolate, at least 70% cocoa solids

1 small orange
3 medium eggs

Place a glass heatproof bowl over a pan so that it sits above the pan without touching the bottom; it should be clear by at least 1 inch. You will also need four small glasses or ramekins.

SERVINGS		NUTRITIONAL INFO	
Carbohydrate	2	Calories	245
Protein	1	Carbohydrate	24 g
Fat	2	Protein	8 g
Dairy	0	Fiber	3 g
Fruit	0	Salt	0.2 g
Vegetables	0		

Break the chocolate into small pieces and put it in the bowl. Zest and juice the orange, then set the zest to one side. Add most of the orange juice to the bowl with the chocolate. Put about ½ inch of water into the pan and bring it to a steady simmer over medium heat. Place the bowl over, but not touching, the water (double-check that it isn't touching the surface) and allow the chocolate to melt, stirring it with a wooden spoon.

Separate the eggs and put the whites in another bowl. Using an electric whisk if possible, whisk the whites until they form soft peaks, by which time the chocolate should have melted. Take the bowl off the pan and add the rest of the orange juice.

Add the egg yolks to the chocolate mixture and beat them in, working energetically. When the egg yolks are all combined and the chocolate has a lovely glossy appearance, add some of the whisked egg white. Using a metal spoon, gently fold it in until the mixture is a uniform color, then repeat until all the white has been added. Now carefully spoon the chocolate mousse into the glasses or ramekins, tap them on the countertop to level them off, and then put them in the refrigerator to chill for at least 5 hours or overnight.

Just before serving, sprinkle some of the reserved orange zest over each one.

Tips:

▶ A few fresh raspberries on the side make a lovely addition.

▶ This healthier version of a classic dish is still deliciously rich (you may find that it will stretch to 6 servings).

▶ It is adaptable: You could use strong black coffee instead of the orange juice, for instance. You'll need about 4 tablespoons in total.

Prune delight
Serves 4

7 oz pitted prunes
1 tbsp clear honey
1 cup (8 oz) low-fat or
fat-free Greek yogurt

SERVINGS		NUTRITIONAL INFO	
Carbohydrate	1	Calories	147
Protein	0	Carbohydrate	29 g
Fat	0	Protein	5 g
Dairy	½	Fiber	4 g
Fruit	1½	Salt	0.1 g
Vegetables	0		

Put the prunes into a bowl and pour a cup of water over them, stir, cover, and set it aside. Soak them overnight or for several hours.

Empty the prunes and their soaking liquid into a pot over high heat and bring them to a boil. Then lower the heat and simmer for about 15 minutes, by which time they should be starting to fall apart. Purée them with a handheld blender or food processor and transfer to a clean bowl; alternatively, push the cooked prunes through a strainer into the bowl with a wooden spoon. Set the prune purée aside and allow it to cool.

Mix the honey and the yogurt together well, then spoon this mixture into the cooled prunes. Stir together thoroughly and then transfer the mixture into a serving bowl or into individual ramekins or glasses. Chill for at least an hour before serving.

Tip:

▶ For a fragrant flavor variation, use a scented tea such as Earl Grey as the soaking liquid.

Apple fool with heather honey
Serves 4

3 large cooking apples
pinch of cinnamon, to taste
* (optional)*
juice of 1 orange
2 tsp heather honey, or
* similarly strongly flavored*
* honey*
10½ oz low-fat or fat-free

Greek yogurt

SERVINGS		NUTRITIONAL INFO	
Carbohydrate	½	Calories	122
Protein	0	Carbohydrate	22 g
Fat	0	Protein	5 g
Dairy	½	Fiber	1 g
Fruit	2	Salt	0.2 g
Vegetables	0		

Peel, core, and chop the apples and put them straight into a pot with a little water—no more than ¼ cup. Add the cinnamon, if using, and the orange juice. Simmer the apples gently until they are really soft, stirring to ensure they don't stick to the bottom of the pan. Remove the pan from the heat and allow the apples to cool down, then blend them until smooth. Spoon the apple purée into a large bowl, cover it with plastic wrap, and chill in the fridge for at least 1 hour.

Once the purée is thoroughly chilled, add the honey and the yogurt. Gently fold these into the apple purée, then spoon it into serving dishes. These can either be served immediately or be put back in the fridge to chill once more and be used later.

Hosaf—Turkish dried fruit salad

Serves 2

6 pitted prunes
6 dried apricots
2 tsp golden raisins
1 tsp pine nuts
1 tsp unsalted pistachios,
  chopped (optional)
1 tbsp slivered almonds

SERVINGS		NUTRITIONAL INFO	
Protein	0	Calories	249
Fat	1½	Carbohydrate	30 g
Dairy	0	Protein	7 g
Fruit	2	Fiber	7 g
Vegetables	0	Salt	<0.1 g

Put the prunes, apricots, raisins, and pine nuts in a small pot, with enough water to just cover everything. Stir well and put the pot on medium heat. Simmer the fruit gently for 20–25 minutes, then empty into a bowl and allow it to cool down for 2 hours (or even overnight). Put the Hosaf into 2 serving dishes and scatter the almonds and pistachios over it just before serving.

Tip:
▶ Traditionally, the pine nuts should be soft. If you prefer them crunchier, add them at the end with the almonds and pistachios.

final word

Some of the Dieters who started The 2-Day Diet had never tried to lose weight before, but many of them had tried over and over again—sometimes losing weight, but mainly putting it back on. Their success with this new diet—which amazed many of them and delighted us—proved to us that there is another way to lose weight and keep it off for good. If you are one of those people, or if you simply want an alternative to the grind of a seven-day diet, The 2-Day Diet can work for you. The formula is a simple one: two days of restricted high-protein/low-carb eating, five days of an unrestricted healthy Mediterranean diet and regular exercise. We know it's not a quick fix and it may take a while for you to adjust your eating habits, but we believe that this is a truly innovative—and healthy—approach to weight loss. We will continue with our research to understand more about the particular health benefits of this diet and this type of weight loss, but in the meantime we hope that The 2-Day Diet will be the approach that works for you. Follow the Diet, get going on an exercise program, and when you've lost your weight, stay with The 1-Day Maintenance Diet and you will achieve the healthy weight and the healthy body you have been hoping for.

appendixes

Appendix A:
How much body fat do I have?

Female Body Fat Percentage Calculator

BMI	Age											
	18	20	25	30	35	40	45	50	55	60	65	70
18	20	20	21	22	23	24	26	27	28	29	30	31
19	22	22	23	24	25	26	27	28	29	30	31	32
20	24	24	25	26	27	28	29	30	31	32	33	33
21	26	26	27	28	29	29	30	31	32	33	34	35
22	27	28	29	29	30	31	32	33	34	34	35	36
23	29	30	30	31	32	33	33	34	35	36	36	37
24	31	31	32	33	33	34	35	36	36	37	38	38
25	33	33	34	34	35	36	36	37	38	38	39	40
26	34	34	35	36	36	37	38	38	39	39	40	41
27	36	36	37	37	38	38	39	39	40	41	41	42
28	37	37	38	39	39	40	40	41	41	42	42	43
29	39	39	39	40	40	41	41	42	42	43	43	44
30	40	40	41	41	42	42	43	43	43	44	44	45
31	41	42	42	42	43	43	44	44	45	45	45	46
32	43	43	43	44	44	44	45	45	46	46	46	47
33	44	44	44	45	45	45	46	46	47	47	47	48
34	45	45	46	46	46	46	47	47	47	48	48	48
35	46	46	47	47	47	47	48	48	48	49	49	49
36	47	47	48	48	48	48	49	49	49	50	50	50
37	48	48	49	49	49	49	50	50	50	50	51	51
38	49	49	50	50	50	50	50	51	51	51	51	52
39	50	50	50	51	51	51	51	51	52	52	52	52
40	51	51	51	51	52	52	52	52	52	53	53	53

To find your body fat percentage, go down to your BMI score and then across to your closest age. You can calculate your BMI on page 31.

For example, a female who has a BMI of 22 and is 42 years old has a body fat percentage of 31%.

Male Body Fat Percentage Calculator

BMI	Age											
	18	20	25	30	35	40	45	50	55	60	65	70
18	11	11	12	13	14	15	16	17	19	20	21	22
19	13	13	14	15	16	17	18	19	20	21	22	23
20	15	15	16	17	18	19	20	21	22	23	24	25
21	17	17	18	19	20	21	22	23	24	24	25	26
22	19	19	20	21	22	23	24	24	25	26	27	28
23	21	21	22	23	24	25	25	26	27	28	28	29
24	23	23	24	25	26	26	27	28	28	29	30	31
25	25	25	26	27	27	28	29	29	30	31	31	32
26	27	27	28	28	29	30	30	31	31	32	33	33
27	29	29	29	30	31	31	32	32	33	34	34	35
28	30	31	31	32	32	33	33	34	34	35	36	36
29	32	32	33	33	34	34	35	35	36	36	37	37
30	34	34	35	35	35	36	36	37	37	38	38	39
31	35	36	36	37	37	37	38	38	39	39	39	40
32	37	37	38	38	38	39	39	40	40	40	41	41
33	39	39	39	39	40	40	41	41	41	42	42	42
34	40	40	41	41	41	42	42	42	43	43	43	44
35	42	42	42	42	43	43	43	44	44	44	44	45
36	43	43	43	44	44	44	45	45	45	45	46	46
37	44	44	45	45	45	45	46	46	46	47	47	47
38	46	46	46	46	47	47	47	47	47	48	48	48
39	47	47	47	48	48	48	48	48	49	49	49	49
40	48	48	49	49	49	49	49	49	50	50	50	50

To find your body fat percentage, go down to your BMI score and then across to your closest age. You can calculate your BMI on page 31.

For example, a male who has a BMI of 22 and is 42 years old has a body fat percentage of 23%.

Body fat calculator based on CUN-BAE equation.[1]

Women should have between 20% and 34% of their body weight as fat, men 8–25%.[2]

Appendix B: How much can I eat on each of my two restricted days?

The food lists below show how much you can eat on each restricted day. If you feel full, you do not have to eat the maximum fat servings. Try to eat the minimum protein and all of your vegetable, dairy, and fruit allowance. For detailed information, including variations for vegetarians, see chapter 3.

Carbohydrate foods	
Carbohydrates are not allowed on the two restricted diet days of The 2-Day Diet.	0 servings

Protein	1 serving equal to:
Women: minimum 4–maximum 12 servings Men: minimum 4–maximum 14 servings	
Fresh or smoked white fish, e.g., flounder or cod	2 oz (two fish-finger-size pieces)
Seafood, e.g., shrimp, mussels, crab	1½ oz
Canned tuna in brine or spring water	1½ oz
Oily fish (fresh or canned) in tomato sauce or oil (drained)—for example, mackerel, sardines, salmon, trout, tuna, smoked salmon* or trout* or kippers*	1 oz
Chicken, turkey, duck, pheasant (cooked without skin)	1 oz (slice the size of a playing card)
Lean beef, pork, lamb, rabbit, venison, organ meats	1 oz (slice the size of a playing card)
Lean bacon*	1 broiled slice
Lean ham*	2 medium slices or 4 wafer-thin slices

* See Salt (page 55).

Protein foods continued	1 serving equal to:
Eggs	1 medium/large egg
Tofu	1¾ oz

Include only *one* of the below on *each* restricted day. They count toward your daily protein allowance.

Protein	Maximum	Servings
Textured vegetable protein (TVP)	maximum 1 oz per day	3
Soy and edamame beans	maximum 2 oz per day	2
Low-fat hummus	maximum 1 tablespoon (½ oz) per day	1
Quorn	maximum 4 oz per day	4

Fat	Serving equal to:
Women: maximum 5 servings Men: maximum 6 servings	
Margarine or low-fat spread (avoid the "buttery" types)	1 teaspoon
Olive oil or other oil (not palm, coconut, or ghee)	2 teaspoons
Oil-based dressing	2 teaspoons
Unsalted or salted* or dry roasted nuts (not honey roast)	2 teaspoons per serving or 3 walnut halves, 3 Brazil nuts, 4 almonds, 8 peanuts, 10 cashews, or 10 pistachios (not chestnuts)
Pesto	1 teaspoon
Mayonnaise	1 teaspoon
Low-fat mayonnaise	1 tablespoon
Olives*	10
Almond or cashew butter	1 teaspoon

* See Salt (page 55).

You can only have one of the following fatty foods on each restricted day, as they contain some carbohydrate. They count toward your fat serving allowance.

Fat	Maximum	Servings
Avocado	½ pear	2
Guacamole	2 tablespoons	2
Low-fat guacamole	2 tablespoons	1

Dairy (3 servings per day for all)	1 serving equal to:
Milk (1% or fat-free)	1 cup (8 oz)
Soy or almond milk (unsweetened with added calcium)	1 cup (8 oz)
Yogurt: diet fruit, plain soy; Greek, plain (all low-fat)	1 small container (4–5 oz) or 3 heaping tablespoons
Whole-milk plain yogurt	2 heaping tablespoons
Cottage cheese (low-fat)	2 tablespoons (2½ oz)
Cream cheese (light or extra-light)	1 tablespoon (1 oz)
Lower-fat cheeses: low-fat cheddar, Edam, feta, Camembert, ricotta, mozzarella, halloumi	Matchbox size—1 oz per serving to a maximum of 4 oz for women per week and 5 oz for men on restricted and unrestricted days

Vegetables (5 servings per day for all)	1 serving equal to 2½ oz
Artichoke	2 globe hearts
Asparagus, canned	7 spears
Asparagus, fresh	5 spears
Beans, broad	4 heaping tablespoons
Beans, string	4 heaping tablespoons

Vegetables continued	1 serving equal to 2½ oz
Bean sprouts, fresh	2 handfuls
Broccoli	2 spears
Brussels sprouts	8
Cabbage	⅙ small cabbage or 3 heaping tablespoons shredded leaves
Cauliflower	8 florets
Celeriac	3 heaping tablespoons
Celery	3 sticks
Chinese cabbage	⅕ "head"
Corn, baby (whole, not kernels)	6
Cucumber	2-in piece
Curly kale, cooked	4 heaping tablespoons
Eggplant	⅓ medium
Fennel	½ cup sliced
Karela or gourd	½
Leeks	1 medium
Lettuce (mixed leaves or arugula)	2⅓ cups
Mushrooms, fresh	14 button or 3 handfuls of slices
Mushrooms, dried	2 tablespoons or handful porcini
Okra	16 medium
Pak choi	2 handfuls
Pepper (green only)	½
Pumpkin	3 heaping tablespoons
Radish	10
Scallions	8

Vegetables continued	1 serving equal to 2½ oz
Snow peas	1 handful
Spinach, cooked	2 heaping tablespoons
Spinach, fresh	2⅓ cups
Spring greens, cooked	4 heaping tablespoons
Tomato, canned	2 plum tomatoes or ½ can chopped
Tomato, fresh	1 medium or 7 cherry
Tomato purée	1 heaping tablespoon
Tomato, sun-dried	4 pieces
Watercress	1 cereal bowlful
Zucchini	½ large

Fruit (1 servings per day for all)	1 serving equal to 2½ oz
Apricots	3 fresh or dried
Blackberries	1 handful
Blackcurrants	4 heaping tablespoons
Redcurrants	4 heaping tablespoons
Grapefruit	½ whole fruit
Melon	2-in slice
Papaya	1 slice
Pineapple	1 large slice
Raspberries	2 handfuls
Strawberries	7
Stewed rhubarb or cranberries, with sweetener	3 heaping tablespoons

Flavorings	
Lemon juice; fresh or dried herbs; spices; black pepper; mustard; horseradish; vinegars; garlic, fresh or pre-chopped; chili, fresh or dried; soy sauce; miso paste; fish sauce; Worcestershire sauce	Unlimited

Drinks	At least 8 drinks or 2 quarts a day
Water (still or sparkling)	Unlimited
Tea and coffee, caffeinated or decaffeinated	Unlimited
Fruit, herbal, or green teas	Unlimited
Sugar-free or diet fruit drinks or carbonated drinks	Up to a maximum of 8 12-oz cans (3 quarts) per week

Appendix C: How much can I eat on each unrestricted day of The 2-Day Diet?

We encourage you to follow a healthy Mediterranean diet on your unrestricted days. This allows you a wider range of foods than your two restricted days and includes carbohydrates, protein, low-fat dairy foods, and a wide range of fruits and vegetables. The tables below are a guide to what makes up a single serving of a given food. You are allowed different numbers of servings from each food group, depending on your gender, weight, and age. The tables in Appendix D will advise the right quantity of these servings for you. For detailed information on the Mediterranean diet please refer to chapter 4.

Carbohydrate foods (amounts vary—check Appendix D)	1 serving equal to:
Whole wheat or oat breakfast cereal	3 level tablespoons (¾ oz), or 2 biscuits shredded wheat
Steel-cut oats or sugar-free muesli	1 heaping tablespoon (⅔ oz)
Whole grain, whole wheat, rye	Medium slice, ½ roll
Pita bread, chapati, tortilla wrap (whole wheat or multigrain versions)	½ large
Rye crisps	2
Whole wheat cracker	2
Dried whole wheat pasta or brown rice	1 tablespoon uncooked (1 oz) or 2 tablespoons cooked (2 oz)
Couscous, bulgur wheat, pearl barley, quinoa	1 tablespoon uncooked (1 oz) or 2 tablespoons cooked (2 oz)
Lasagne (preferably whole wheat)	1 sheet
Noodles (preferably whole wheat)	Half a dried block or nest (1¾ oz)
Baked or boiled potato (in skin)	1 small (4 oz) raw weight

Carbohydrate foods continued	1 serving equal to:
Yam, sweet potato	1 small (3 oz) raw weight
Whole wheat pizza crust	⅙ of thin medium pizza base
Corn	½ corn on the cob or 2 tablespoons kernels
Whole wheat flour	Level tablespoon
Popcorn	⅔ oz

Protein foods (amounts vary—check Appendix D)	1 serving equal to:
Fresh or smoked* white fish (for example, trout or cod)	2 oz (two fish-finger-size pieces)
Canned tuna in brine or spring water	1½ oz
Oily fish (fresh or canned) in tomato sauce or oil (drained)—for example, mackerel, sardines, salmon, trout, tuna, smoked salmon* or trout* or kippers*	1 oz
Seafood—e.g., shrimp, mussels, crab	1½ oz
Chicken, turkey, or duck (cooked without the skin)	1 oz (a slice the size of a playing card)
Lean beef, pork, lamb, rabbit, venison, or organ meats (fat removed)	1 oz per serving to a maximum of 1 lb 1 oz per week for women and 1 lb 4 oz per week for men
Lean bacon*	1 slice
Eggs	1 medium/large
Ham*	2 medium slices or 4 wafer-thin slices
Baked beans	2 level tablespoons (2 oz)
Lentils, chickpeas, and beans	1 tablespoon (⅔ oz) raw or 1½ tablespoons cooked or canned (2 oz)

* Try to have these salty foods only once during your five unrestricted days.

Protein foods continued	1 serving equal to:
Quorn—e.g., pieces, ground, fillets	1 oz
Vegetarian sausage	½
Tofu	⅛ of package (1¾ oz)
Textured vegetable protein (TVP)	1 heaping tablespoon (⅓ oz) uncooked
Frozen vegetarian mince	1 oz
Low-fat hummus	1 level tablespoon (1 oz)

Fat (amounts vary according to sex, age and weight—check Appendix D)	1 serving equal to:
Margarine or low-fat spread (avoid the buttery types)	1 teaspoon
Olive oil or other oil	2 teaspoons
Oil-based dressing	2 teaspoons
Unsalted nuts/seeds	2 teaspoons or 3 walnut halves, 3 Brazil nuts, 4 almonds, 8 peanuts, 10 cashews or pistachios
Avocado	¼ average pear
Pesto	1 level teaspoon
Olives	10
Mayonnaise	1 teaspoon
Guacamole or low-fat mayonnaise	1 tablespoon
Low-fat guacamole	2 tablespoons
Almond or cashew butter	1 heaping teaspoon

Milk and dairy foods (3 servings per day for all)	1 serving is:
Milk (1% or fat-free)	1 cup (8 oz)
Alternative "milks"—e.g., soy, almond (unsweetened)	1 cup (8 oz)
Reduced-fat evaporated milk	1 level tablespoon
Yogurt: diet fruit, plain soy; Greek, plain (all low-fat)	1 5-oz container or 3 heaping tablespoons
Yogurt: low-fat fruit, whole-milk fruit, and plain, flavored soy yogurt	2½–3 oz or 2 heaping tablespoons
Cottage cheese (low-fat)	2 tablespoons
Cream cheese (light or extra-light)	1 level tablespoon (1 oz)
Low-fat or fat-free ricotta	3 level tablespoons (3 oz)
Lower-fat cheeses: Low-fat cheddar, Edam, smoked Gouda, feta, Camembert, mozzarella, low-fat halloumi	Matchbox-size (1 oz). No more than 4 oz per week for women and 5 oz for men.

Vegetables (at least 5 servings per day for all)	1 serving equal to 2½ oz
Any boiled or steamed vegetables (except potato, yam, corn, which are carbohydrates, or beans, which are counted as protein)	2–3 heaping tablespoons
Salad	1 bowl
Homemade vegetable soup	½ cup
Vegetable juice*	1 cup
Tomato purée	1 level tablespoon

* Limit to 1 glass of fruit and vegetable juice per day.

Fruit (2 servings per day for all)	1 serving is:
Banana	1 small
Blackberries, raspberries, strawberries	1 cup (2½ oz)
Canned fruit (in natural juice)	3 level tablespoons
Dried fruit	3 dried apricots/handful raisins
Fruit juice	Small glass (½ cup)*
Grapes, cherries	15
Grapefruit	½ whole fruit
Melon/pineapple/papaya	1 slice
Oranges, pear, apple	1 fruit
Small fruits: clementines, apricots	2 fruits
Stewed fruit (unsweetened or with sweetener)	3 level tablespoons

* Limit to 1 glass of fruit and vegetable juice per day.

Drinks	At least 8 drinks or 2 quarts a day
Water (still or sparkling)	Unlimited
Tea and coffee, caffeinated or decaffeinated	Unlimited
Fruit, herbal, or green teas	Unlimited
Sugar-free or diet fruit drinks or carbonated drinks	Up to a maximum of 8 12-ounce cans per week
Alcohol	Up to a maximum of 7 units a week (see page 87)

Treats (up to 3 servings a week on unrestricted days)	Treat serving:
Low-fat potato chips	1 small package (¾–1 oz)
Plain or chocolate graham crackers or small oatmeal cookies	2
Chocolate (ideally dark 70% cocoa or higher content)	5 small squares or 1 oz
Ice cream	2 scoops standard or 1 scoop premium
Mini cupcakes	2 small cakes with thin or no icing
Granola bar	½ bar
Small chocolate chip cookies	3
Individual chocolate or truffle	3

Appendix D: Quick reference to how much I can eat

Use these tables to look up how many calories or servings of foods you can have a day according to your gender, age, and weight. They include information for both weight loss and weight maintenance.

- Energy requirements have been determined using the Henry equations[3] based on your gender, age, and weight. You will lose weight more quickly if you also follow the exercise recommendations in the book.
- It is important to get adequate protein, dairy, fruit, and vegetables on the two restricted and five unrestricted days of The 2-Day Diet. This is why there are minimum amounts for protein and recommended amounts for dairy, fruit, and vegetables each day. These meal plans have been designed so you will achieve the recommended amount of .6 g of protein per kilogram of body weight each day.[4]
- You do not need to eat the maximum amounts in the table. However, it is important to get the balance of foods right. For example, if you only have two-thirds of your maximum protein servings, you should also roughly aim for two-thirds of your maximum fat and high-fiber carbohydrate servings.
- Try to get 24 g of fiber on each unrestricted day (see page 336).

Weight loss calculator | Males
Up to 175 lb

	2 restricted days	5 unrestricted days														
		Less than 119 lb			119–133 lb			133–147 lb			147–161 lb			161–175 lb		
		Age 18–29	Age 30–60	Age 60+	Age 18–29	Age 30–60	Age 60+	Age 18–29	Age 30–60	Age 60+	Age 18–29	Age 30–60	Age 60+	Age 18–29	Age 30–60	Age 60+
Maximum cal per day	1,100	1,600	1,600	1,400	1,700	1,600	1,400	1,900	1,800	1,600	2,000	1,900	1,700	2,100	2,000	1,800
Carbohydrate servings	0	Max 7	Max 7	Max 6	Max 7	Max 7	Max 6	Max 8	Max 8	Max 7	Max 9	Max 9	Max 7	Max 11	Max 9	Max 8
Protein servings	Min 4	Min 3	Min 3	Min 3	Min 4	Min 4	Min 4	Min 5	Min 5	Min 5	Min 6	Min 6	Min 6	Min 7	Min 7	Min 7
	Max 14	Max 9	Max 9	Max 8	Max 10	Max 9	Max 8	Max 12	Max 11	Max 9	Max 14	Max 12	Max 10	Max 14	Max 14	Max 11
Fat servings	Max 6	Max 4	Max 4	Max 3	Max 5	Max 4	Max 3	Max 5	Max 5	Max 4	Max 5	Max 5	Max 5	Max 5	Max 5	Max 5
Dairy servings	3 (recommended)	3 (recommended for all weight groups)														
Vegetable servings	5 (recommended)	5 (recommended for all weight groups)														
Fruit servings	1 (recommended)	2 (recommended for all weight groups)														

Weight loss calculator | Males

Over 175 lb

	2 restricted days	5 unrestricted days											
		175–189 lb			189–203 lb			203–295 lb			Above 295 lb		
		Age 18–29	Age 30–60	Age 60+	Age 18–29	Age 30–60	Age 60+	Age 18–29	Age 30–60	Age 60+	Age 18–29	Age 30–60	Age 60+
Maximum cal per day	1,100	2,300	2,200	2,000	2,500	2,300	2,100	2,500	2,400	2,200	2,500	2,500	2,300
Carbohydrate servings	0	Max 12	Max 11	Max 9	Max 13	Max 12	Max 11	Max 13	Max 12	Max 11	Max 13	Max 13	Max 12
Protein servings	Min 4	Min 8	Min 8	Min 8	Min 9	Min 9	Min 9	Min 10	Min 10	Min 10	Min 11	Min 11	Min 11
	Max 14	Max 16	Max 15	Max 14	Max 17	Max 16	Max 14	Max 17	Max 17	Max 15	Max 17	Max 17	Max 16
Fat servings	Max 6	Max 6	Max 5	Max 5	Max 7	Max 6	Max 5	Max 7	Max 6	Max 5	Max 7	Max 7	Max 6
Dairy servings	3 (recommended)	3 (recommended for all weight groups)											
Vegetable servings	5 (recommended)	5 (recommended for all weight groups)											
Fruit servings	1 (recommended)	2 (recommended for all weight groups)											

Weight loss calculator | Females
Up to 175 lb

	2 restricted days	5 unrestricted days														
		Less than 119 lb			119–133 lb			133–147 lb			147–161 lb			161–175 lb		
		Age 18–29	Age 30–60	Age 60+	Age 18–29	Age 30–60	Age 60+	Age 18–29	Age 30–60	Age 60+	Age 18–29	Age 30–60	Age 60+	Age 18–29	Age 30–60	Age 60+
Maximum cal per day	1,000	1,500	1,400	1,400	1,500	1,400	1,400	1,700	1,500	1,400	1,800	1,600	1,500	1,900	1,700	1,600
Carbohydrate servings	0	Max 6	Max 6	Max 6	Max 6	Max 6	Max 6	Max 7	Max 6	Max 6	Max 8	Max 7	Max 6	Max 9	Max 7	Max 7
Protein servings	Min 4	Min 3	Min 3	Min 3	Min 4	Min 4	Min 4	Min 5	Min 5	Min 5	Min 6	Min 6	Min 6	Min 7	Min 7	Min 7
	Max 12	Max 8	Max 8	Max 8	Max 8	Max 8	Max 8	Max 10	Max 8	Max 8	Max 11	Max 9	Max 8	Max 12	Max 10	Max 9
Fat servings	Max 5	Max 4	Max 3	Max 3	Max 4	Max 3	Max 3	Max 5	Max 4	Max 3	Max 5	Max 4	Max 4	Max 5	Max 5	Max 4
Dairy servings	3 (recommended)	3 (recommended for all weight groups)														
Vegetable servings	5 (recommended)	5 (recommended for all weight groups)														
Fruit servings	1 (recommenced)	2 (recommended for all weight groups)														

Weight loss calculator | Females
Over 175 lb

	2 restricted days	5 unrestricted days											
		175–189 lb			189–203 lb			203–217 lb			Above 217 lb		
		Age 18–29	Age 30–60	Age 60+	Age 18–29	Age 30–60	Age 60+	Age 18–29	Age 30–60	Age 60+	Age 18–29	Age 30–60	Age 60+
Maximum cal per day	1,000	2,000	1,800	1,700	2,000	1,900	1,300	2,000	2,000	1,800	2,000	2,000	1,900
Carbohydrate servings	0	Max 9	Max 8	Max 7	Max 9	Max 9	Max 8	Max 9	Max 9	Max 8	Max 9	Max 9	Max 9
Protein servings	Min 4	Min 8	Min 8	Min 8	Min 9	Min 9	Min 9	Min 10	Min 10	Min 10	Min 11	Min 11	Min 11
	Max 12	Max 14	Max 11	Max 10	Max 14	Max 12	Max 11	Max 14	Max 14	Max 11	Max 14	Max 14	Max 12
Fat servings	Max 5	Max 5	Max 5	Max 5	Max 5	Max 5	Max 5	Max 5	Max 5	Max 5	Max 5	Max 5	Max 5
Dairy servings	3 (recommended)	3 (recommended for all weight groups)											
Vegetable servings	5 (recommended)	5 (recommended for all weight groups)											
Fruit servings	1 (recommended)	2 (recommended for all weight groups)											

Weight maintenance calculator | Males
Up to 161 lb

	1 restricted days	6 unrestricted days											
		Less than 119 lb			119–133 lb			133–147 lb			147–161 lb		
		Age 18–29	Age 30–60	Age 60+	Age 18–29	Age 30–60	Age 60+	Age 18–29	Age 30–60	Age 60+	Age 18–29	Age 30–60	Age 60+
Maximum cal per day	1,100	1,900	1,800	1,600	2,000	1,900	1,700	2,100	2,000	1,800	2,300	2,200	2,000
Carbohydrate servings	0	Max 8	Max 8	Max 7	Max 9	Max 9	Max 7	Max 11	Max 9	Max 8	Max 12	Max 11	Max 9
Protein servings	Min 4	Min 3	Min 3	Min 3	Min 4	Min 4	Min 4	Min 5	Min 5	Min 5	Min 6	Min 6	Min 6
	Max 14	Max 12	Max 11	Max 9	Max 14	Max 12	Max 10	Max 14	Max 14	Max 11	Max 16	Max 15	Max 14
Fat servings	Max 6	Max 5	Max 5	Max 4	Max 5	Max 5	Max 5	Max 5	Max 5	Max 5	Max 6	Max 5	Max 5
Dairy servings	3 (recommended)	3 (recommended for all weight groups)											
Vegetable servings	5 (recommended)	5 (recommended for all weight groups)											
Fruit servings	1 (recommended)	2 (recommended for all weight groups)											

Weight maintenance calculator | Males
Over 161 lb

	1 restricted days	6 unrestricted days												
		161–175 lb			175–189 lb			189–203 lb			Above 203 lb			
		Age 18–29	Age 30–60	Age 60+	Age 18–29	Age 30–60	Age 60+	Age 18–29	Age 30–60	Age 60+	Age 18–29	Age 30–60	Age 60+	
Maximum cal per day	1,100	2,400	2,300	2,100	2,500	2,400	2,200	2,500	2,500	2,300	2,500	2,500	2,500	
Carbohydrate servings	0	Max 12	Max 12	Max 11	Max 13	Max 12	Max 11	Max 13	Max 13	Max 12	Max 13	Max 13	Max 13	
Protein servings	Min 4	Min 7	Min 7	Min 7	Min 8	Min 8	Min 8	Min 9	Min 9	Min 9	Min 10	Min 10	Min 10	
	Max 14	Max 17	Max 16	Max 14	Max 17	Max 17	Max 15	Max 17	Max 17	Max 16	Max 17	Max 17	Max 17	
Fat servings	Max 6	Max 6	Max 6	Max 5	Max 7	Max 6	Max 5	Max 7	Max 7	Max 6	Max 7	Max 7	Max 7	
Dairy servings	3 (recommended)	3 (recommended for all weight groups)												
Vegetable servings	5 (recommended)	5 (recommended for all weight groups)												
Fruit servings	1 (recommended)	2 (recommended for all weight groups)												

Weight maintenance calculator | Females
Up to 161 lb

	1 restricted days	6 unrestricted days — Less than 119 lb, Age 18–29	Age 30–60	Age 60+	119–133 lb, Age 18–29	Age 30–60	Age 60+	133–147 lb, Age 18–29	Age 30–60	Age 60+	147–161 lb, Age 18–29	Age 30–60	Age 60+
Maximum cal per day	1,000	1,700	1,600	1,500	1,800	1,700	1,500	1,900	1,800	1,600	2,000	1,900	1,700
Carbohydrate servings	0	Max 7	Max 7	Max 6	Max 8	Max 7	Max 6	Max 9	Max 8	Max 7	Max 9	Max 9	Max 7
Protein servings	Min 4	Min 3	Min 3	Min 3	Min 4	Min 4	Min 4	Min 5	Min 5	Min 5	Min 6	Min 6	Min 6
	Max 12	Max 10	Max 9	Max 8	Max 11	Max 10	Max 8	Max 12	Max 11	Max 9	Max 14	Max 12	Max 10
Fat servings	Max 5	Max 5	Max 4	Max 4	Max 5	Max 5	Max 4	Max 5	Max 5	Max 4	Max 5	Max 5	Max 5
Dairy servings	3 (recommended)	3 (recommended for all weight groups)											
Vegetable servings	5 (recommended)	5 (recommended for all weight groups)											
Fruit servings	1 (recommended)	2 (recommended for all weight groups)											

Weight maintenance calculator | Females

Over 161 lb

	1 restricted days	6 unrestricted days											
		161–175 lb			175–189 lb			189–203 lb			Above 203 lb		
		Age 18–29	Age 30–60	Age 60+	Age 18–29	Age 30–60	Age 60+	Age 18–29	Age 30–60	Age 60+	Age 18–29	Age 30–60	Age 60+
Maximum cal per day	1,000	2,000	1,900	1,800	2,000	2,000	1,900	2,000	2,000	2,000	2,000	2,000	2,000
Carbohydrate servings	0	Max 9	Max 9	Max 8	Max 9	Max 9	Max 9	Max 9	Max 9	Max 9	Max 9	Max 9	Max 9
Protein servings	Min 4	Min 7	Min 7	Min 7	Min 8	Min 8	Min 8	Min 9	Min 9	Min 9	Min 10	Min 10	Min 10
	Max 12	Max 14	Max 12	Max 11	Max 14	Max 14	Max 12	Max 14	Max 14	Max 14	Max 14	Max 14	Max 14
Fat servings	Max 5	Max 5	Max 5	Max 5	Max 5	Max 5	Max 5	Max 5	Max 5	Max 5	Max 5	Max 5	Max 5
Dairy servings	3 (recommended)	3 (recommended for all weight groups)											
Vegetable servings	5 (recommended)	5 (recommended for all weight groups)											
Fruit servings	1 (recommended)	2 (recommended for all weight groups)											

Appendix E: Top 10 fiber-rich foods

The two tables below show the top 10 fiber-rich foods for your restricted and unrestricted days.[5, 6] Aim to include as many as possible within your servings allowance.

Food	Serving size description	g	Total fiber (g)	Soluble fiber (g)	Insoluble fiber (g)
Restricted days					
Raspberries	1 handful	80	5.5	1.5	4.0
Frozen soybeans	4 tbsp	60	3.7	1.8	1.9
Green beans	4 tbsp	80	2.5	0.6	1.9
Broccoli	2 spears	80	2.4	1.2	1.2
Apricots, dried	3	25	2.2	1.2	1.0
Cauliflower	8 florets	80	2.2	0.9	1.3
Spinach (cooked)	2 tbsp	80	2.2	0.7	1.5
Brussels sprouts	8	80	2.1	1.1	1.0
Flaxseeds	2 tsp	7	1.9	0.6	1.3
Almonds	4 nuts	8	0.8	0.1	0.7
Unrestricted days					
High-fiber bran cereal	3 tbsp	24	5.9	1.0	4.9
Raspberries	1 handful	80	5.5	1.5	4.0
Peas	3 tbsp	80	5.4	1.6	3.8
Kidney beans	1 tbsp	40	3.2	0.8	2.4
Bran flakes	3 tbsp	24	3.1	0.3	2.9
Rye crisps	2	20	3.1	1.3	1.8
Pearl barley	Level tbsp uncooked	20	3.1	0.8	2.3
Figs, ready to eat	3	25	3.0	1.4	1.6
Grape-Nuts	3 tbsp	24	2.8	0.8	2.0
Pasta, whole wheat, cooked	2 tbsp	60	2.8	0.6	2.2

Appendix F: How to include more daily physical activity

The chart below shows how you can burn off more calories during the day by simply making some small adjustments to your normal routine. You should aim to combine planned exercise with small amounts of activity during the day for the best results.

Gym day with minimal daily activities	Calories used *	Non-gym day with daily activities	Calories used*
Take the bus to work (20 min)	30	Get off the bus 5 min early and walk 15 min	84
Take the elevator up 2 floors, 5 times during the day	3	Walk up and down 2 floors, 5 times during the day	54
E-mail a colleague	8	Walk 2 min to colleague, stand and talk 5 min, walk 2 min back to desk	33
Buy sandwich from cart	3	Walk to sandwich shop, 5 min each way	35
Take the bus home (20 min)	30	Get off the bus 5 min early and walk 15 min	84
Drive to gym (7 min)	20		
Aerobics class (45 min)	262	Watch television (1 hour)	90
Drive home (7 min)	20		
Reheat frozen meal (5 min)	5	Prepare a meal (30 min)	70
Watch television (1 hour 25 min)	128	Vacuum (30 min), iron (30 min)	178
Do online food shopping (30 min)	26	Walk to the shops (15 min each way) Food shopping (30 min)	193
Let the dog out in the yard	2	Walk the dog (30 min)	105
Reading (1 hour 15 min)	115	Reading (15 min)	23
Total calories	652	Total calories	949

*Estimated for a 154 lb woman

Appendix G:
My 12-week exercise plan

This 12-week walking program is designed so you can build up the level of exercise over several weeks. If the first week feels too easy, start at Week 3 or 4; if you're finding it tough, repeat that week until you're ready to move on. Work through the full 12 weeks.

By Week 12 you will be doing 150 minutes of moderate exercise, which is about half an hour for five days a week—irrespective of wherever you were at the start. Moderate exercise walking pace is defined as between 2½ to 4 miles per hour on flat, level ground.

Week		1	2	3	4	5	6	7	8	9	10	11	12
Beginner Not currently exercising at all	Time (min)	5	5	5	10	10	15	15	20	20	25	25	30
	Speed (mph)	1.5	1.5	1.5	1.5	2	2	2	2	2	2	2.5	2.5
	Frequency (sessions/week)	1	2	3	3	3	4	4	4	5	5	5	5
Intermediate Currently doing at least one exercise session a week	Time (min)	10	10	10	15	15	20	20	25	25	30	30	30
	Speed (mph)	2	2	2.5	2.5	2.5	2.5	2.5	3	3	3	3	3
	Frequency (sessions/week)	2	3	3	4	4	4	5	5	5	5	5	5
Advanced Currently doing at least two exercise sessions a week	Time (min)	15	15	15	20	20	20	25	25	30	30	30	30
	Speed (mph)	3	3	3	3	3	3.5	3.5	3.5	3.5	3.5	4	4
	Frequency (sessions/week)	3	4	4	4	5	5	5	5	5	5	5	5

It is recommended that you continue to exercise for 150 minutes per week at a moderate level for another 12 weeks and really get the exercise habit established before you begin to build to 300 minutes of moderate exercise per week.

FurtherInformation

The 2-Day Diet website
www.the2daydietbook.com

Healthy lifestyle information
Healthy People 2020 (science-based national objectives for improving the health of all Americans):
http://www.healthypeople.gov/2020/default.aspx
US Department of Health and Human Services Healthfinder (information and tools to help you and those you care about stay healthy):
http://healthfinder.gov/Default.aspx

Health conditions information
Genesis Breast Cancer Prevention research:
www.genesisuk.org
National Cancer Institute
Breast cancer: http://www.cancer.gov/cancertopics/types/breast
American Heart Association:
www.americanheart.org
American Diabetes Association:
www.diabetes.org
Arthritis Foundation:
www.arthritis.org

Journal resources
PubMed electronic journal resource:
www.ncbi.nlm.nih.gov/entrez

Centers for Disease Control and Prevention:
    www.cdc.gov/Publications
The New England Journal of Medicine:
    www.nejm.org
US Health Statistics:
    CDC/National Center for Health Statistics:
    www.cdc.gov/nchs
MedlinePlus:
    www.nlm.nih.gov/medlineplus/healthstatistics.html

Food

U.S. Food and Drug Administration:
    www.fda.gov/Food/default.htm
Nutrition.gov:
    www.nutrition.gov

Weight Management

Academy of Nutrition and Dietetics:
    www.eatright.org
CDC Division of Nutrition, Physical Activity and Obesity:
    www.cdc.gov/obesity/
National Heart, Lung and Blood Institute guidelines on
    weight management: Identification, Evaluation, Treatment
    of Overweight and Obesity in Adults:
    www.nhlbi.nih.gov/guidelines/obesity/ob_home.htm

Physical Activity

Let's Move!:
    www.letsmove.gov
Every Body Walk!:
    http://everybodywalk.org

President's Council on Fitness, Sports, and Nutrition: www.fitness.gov

Public Health Agency of Canada/Physical Activity: www.phac-aspc.gc.ca/hp-ps/hl-mvs/pa-ap/index-eng.php

For activities or organizations near you, search the Web.

references

1. Why The 2-Day Diet works

1. Harvie M, Howell A, et al., "Association of gain and loss of weight before and after menopause with risk of postmenopausal breast cancer in the Iowa women's health study," *Cancer Epidemiology, Biomarkers & Prevention*, 14/3 (2005), 656–61.

2. Wing RR et al., "Long-term weight loss maintenance," *The American Journal of Clinical Nutrition*, 82/1 Suppl (2005), 222S–225S.

3. www.cdc.gov/obesity/data/adult.html.

4. http://today.duke.edu/2010/10/workobese.html.

5. Cleary MP et al., "Weight-cycling decreases incidence and increases latency of mammary tumors to a greater extent than does chronic caloric restriction in mouse mammary tumor virus-transforming growth factor-alpha female mice," *Cancer Epidemiology, Biomarkers & Prevention*, 11/9 (2002), 836–43.

6. Anson RM, Mattson MP, et al., "Intermittent fasting dissociates beneficial effects of dietary restriction on glucose metabolism and neuronal resistance to injury from calorie intake," *Proceedings of the National Academy of Sciences of the United States of America*, 100/10 (2003), 6216–20.

7. Harvie MN, Howell A, et al., "The effects of intermittent or continuous energy restriction on weight loss and metabolic disease risk markers: a randomized trial in young overweight women," *International Journal of Obesity* (London), 35/5 (2011), 714–27.

8. Harvie MN, Howell A, et al., P3–09–02: "Intermittent Dietary Carbohydrate Restriction Enables Weight Loss and Reduces Breast Cancer Risk Biomarkers," Thirty-Fourth Annual CTRC-AACR San Antonio Breast Cancer Symposium (San Antonio, TX) (Dec 6–10, 2011).

9. Veldhorst MA et al., "Presence or absence of carbohydrates and the proportion of fat in a high-protein diet affect appetite suppression but not energy expenditure in normal-weight human subjects fed in energy balance," *British Journal of Nutrition*, 104/9 (2010), 1395–1405.

10. Johnson F et al., "Dietary restraint and self-regulation in eating behavior," *International Journal of Obesity* (London), 36/5 (2012), 665–74.

11. Jacobsen SC et al., "Effects of short-term high-fat overfeeding on genome-wide DNA methylation in the skeletal muscle of healthy young men," *Diabetologia*, 12 (2012), 3341–49.

12. Timmers S et al., "Calorie restriction-like effects of 30 days of resveratrol supplementation on energy metabolism and metabolic profile in obese humans," *Cell Metabolism*, 14/5 (2011), 612–22.

13. Peeters A et al., "Obesity in adulthood and its consequences for life expectancy: a life-table analysis," *Annals of Internal Medicine*, 138/1 (2003), 24–32.

14. http://www.washingtonpost.com/wp-srv/special/health/healthy/life-expectancy/.

15. Carlson O et al., "Impact of reduced meal frequency without caloric restriction on glucose regulation in healthy, normal-weight middle-aged men and women," *Metabolism*, 56/12 (2007), 1729–34.

16. Sandholt CH et al., "Beyond the fourth wave of genome-wide obesity association studies," *Nutrition & Diabetes*, 2/e37 (2012).

17. Garaulet M et al., "CLOCK gene is implicated in weight reduction in obese patients participating in a dietary programme based on the Mediterranean diet," *International Journal of Obesity* (London), 34/3 (2010), 516–23.

18. Matsuo T et al., "Effects of FTO genotype on weight loss and metabolic risk factors in response to calorie restriction among Japanese women," *Obesity* (Silver Spring), 20/5 (2012), 1122–26.

19. Lovelady C., "Balancing exercise and food intake with lactation to promote post-partum weight loss," *Proceedings of the Nutrition Society*, 70/2 (2011), 181–84.

20. http://www.ncbi.nlm.nih.gov/pubmed.

2. Do I need to lose weight?

1. Shea JL et al., "Body fat percentage is associated with cardiometabolic dysregulation in BMI-defined normal weight subjects," *Nutrition, Metabolism & Cardiovascular Diseases*, 22/9 (2012), 741–47.

2. Sternfeld B et al., "Changes over 14 years in androgenicity and body mass index in a biracial cohort of reproductive-age women," *The Journal of Clinical Endocrinology & Metabolism*, 93/6 (2008), 2158–65.

3. Harvie MN, Howell AH et al., "Central obesity and breast cancer risk: a systematic review," *Obesity Reviews*, 4/3 (2003), 157–73.

4. Beck RJ et al., "Choral singing, performance perception, and immune system changes in salivary immunoglobulin A and cortisol," *Music Perception*, 18 (1999), 87–106.

5. Nackers LM et al., "The association between rate of initial weight loss and long-term success in obesity treatment: does slow and steady win the race?" *International Journal of Behavioral Medicine*, 17/3 (2010), 161–67.

6.   Paulweber B et al., "A European evidence-based guideline for the prevention of type 2 diabetes," *Hormone and Metabolic Research*, 42 Suppl 1 (2010), S3–36.

7.   Maruthur NM et al., "Lifestyle interventions reduce coronary heart disease risk: results from the PREMIER Trial," *Circulation*, 119/15 (2009), 2026–31.

8.   Harvie MN, Howell A et al., "Association of gain and loss of weight before and after menopause with risk of postmenopausal breast cancer in the Iowa women's health study," *Cancer Epidemiology, Biomarkers & Prevention*, 14/3 (2005), 656–61.

9.   Larson-Meyer DE et al., "Effect of calorie restriction with or without exercise on insulin sensitivity, beta-cell function, fat cell size, and ectopic lipid in overweight subjects," *Diabetes Care*, 29/6 (2006), 1337–44.

3. How to do the two restricted days

1.   Pearce KL et al., "Egg consumption as part of an energy-restricted high-protein diet improves blood lipid and blood glucose profiles in individuals with type 2 diabetes," *British Journal of Nutrition*, 105/4 (2011), 584–92.

2.   Lieberman HR et al., "A double-blind, placebo-controlled test of 2 d of calorie deprivation: effects on cognition, activity, sleep, and interstitial glucose concentrations," *The American Journal of Clinical Nutrition*, 88/3 (2008), 667–76.

3.   Brinkworth GD et al., "Long-term effects of a very low-carbohydrate diet and a low-fat diet on mood and cognitive function," *Archives of Internal Medicine*, 169/20 (2009), 1873–80.

4.   Krikorian R et al., "Dietary ketosis enhances memory in mild cognitive impairment," *Neurobiology Aging*, 33/2 (2012), 425–27.

4. How to eat on the five unrestricted days

1.   Willett WC, "The Mediterranean Diet: Science and practice," *Public Health Nutrition*, 9/1A (2006), 105–10.

2.   Sevastianova K et al., "Effect of short-term carbohydrate overfeeding and long-term weight loss on liver fat in overweight humans," *The American Journal of Clinical Nutrition*, 96/4 (2012), 727–34.

3.   Bofetta J et al., "Fruit and vegetable intake and overall cancer risk in the European Prospective Investigation into Cancer and Nutrition (EPIC)," *Journal of the National Cancer Institute*, 102/8 (2010), 529–37.

4.   Houchins JA et al., "Effects of fruit and vegetable, consumed in solid vs. beverage forms, on acute and chronic appetitive responses in lean and obese adults," *International Journal of Obesity* (London) (Nov. 20, 2012).

5.   Stookey JD et al., "Drinking water is associated with weight loss in overweight dieting women independent of diet and activity," *Obesity* (Silver Spring), 16/11 (2008), 2481–88.

6.   Flood-Obbagy JE et al., "The effect of fruit in different forms on energy intake and satiety at a meal," *Appetite*, 52/2 (2009), 416–22.

7.   Backhed F, "Host responses to the human microbiome," *Nutrition Reviews*, 70 Suppl 1 (2012), S14–S17.

8.   http://www.dh.gov.uk/health/2012/06/sodium-intakes/.

9.   Aune D, "Soft drinks, aspartame and the risk of cancer and cardio-vascular disease," *The American Journal of Clinical Nutrition*, 96/6 (2012), 1249–51.

10.   Chapman CD et al., "Lifestyle determinants of the drive to eat: a meta-analysis," *The American Journal of Clinical Nutrition*, 96/3 (2012), 492–97.

11.   Chobanian AV et al., "Seventh report of the Joint National Committee on Prevention, Detection, Evaluation, and Treatment of High Blood Pressure," *Hypertension*, 42/6 (2003), 1206–52.

12.   Nawrot P et al., "Effects of caffeine on human health," *Food Additives and Contaminants*, 20/1 (2003), 1–30.

13.   Almoosawi S et al., "The effect of polyphenol-rich dark chocolate on fasting capillary whole blood glucose, total cholesterol, blood pressure and glucocorticoids in healthy overweight and obese subjects," *British Journal of Nutrition*, 103/6 (2010), 842–850.

5. Making The 2-Day Diet work

1.   Wansink B, "Environmental factors that unknowingly influence the consumption and intake of consumers," *Annual Review of Nutrition*, 24 (2004), 455–79.

2.   Dennis EA et al., "Water consumption increases weight loss during a hypocaloric diet intervention in middle-aged and older adults," *Obesity* (Silver Spring), 18/2 (2010), 300–7.

3.   Rolls BJ et al., "The effect of large portion sizes on energy intake is sustained for 11 days," *Obesity*, 15/6 (2007), 1535–43.

4.   Rolls BJ et al., "Reductions in portion size and energy density of foods are additive and lead to sustained decreases in energy intake," *The American Journal of Clinical Nutrition*, 83/1 (2006), 11–7.

5.   Bellisle F, "Cognitive restraint can be offset by distraction, leading to increased meal intake in women," *The American Journal of Clinical Nutrition*, 74/2 (2001), 197–200.

6.   Hirsch AR et al., "Effect of Television Viewing on Sensory-Specific Satiety: Are Leno and Letterman Obesogenic?" 89th Annual Meeting Endocrine Society (Abstract) (2007).

7. Byrne NM et al., "Does metabolic compensation explain the majority of less-than-expected weight loss in obese adults during a short-term severe diet and exercise intervention?" *International Journal of Obesity*, 36/11 (2012), 1472–78.

8. Bellisle F et al., "Meal frequency and energy balance," *British Journal of Nutrition*, 77/1 (1997), S57–70.

9. Holmback U et al., "The human body may buffer small differences in meal size and timing during a 24-hour wake period provided energy balance is maintained," *Journal of Nutrition*, 133/9 (2003), 2748–55.

10. Nedeltcheva AV et al., "Sleep curtailment is accompanied by increased intake of calories from snacks," *The American Journal of Clinical Nutrition*, 89 (2009), 126–33.

11. Buxton OM et al., "Adverse metabolic consequences in humans of prolonged sleep restriction combined with circadian disruption," *Science Translational Medicine*, 4/129 (2012), 12.

12. Morgan PJ et al., "Efficacy of a workplace-based weight loss program for overweight male shift workers: the Workplace POWER (Preventing Obesity Without Eating like a Rabbit) randomized controlled trial," *Preventive Medicine*, 52/5 (2011), 317–25.

13. Halsey LG et al., "Does consuming breakfast influence activity levels? An experiment into the effect of breakfast consumption on eating habits and energy expenditure," *Public Health Nutrition*, 15/2 (2012), 238–45.

14. Ratliff J et al., "Consuming eggs for breakfast influences plasma glucose and ghrelin, while reducing energy intake during the next 24 hours in adult men," *Nutrition Research*, 30/2 (2010), 96–1003.

15. Mason C et al., "History of weight cycling does not impede future weight loss or metabolic improvements in postmenopausal women," *Metabolism*, 62/1 (2013), 127–36.

16. Smeets AJ et al., "Acute effects on metabolism and appetite profile of one meal difference in the lower range of meal frequency," *British Journal of Nutrition*, 99/6 (2008), 1316–21.

17. Wing RR et al., "Prescribed 'breaks' as a means to disrupt weight control efforts," *Obesity Research*, 11/2 (2003), 287–91.

18. May et al., "Elaborated intrusion theory: a cognitive-emotional theory of food craving," *Current Obesity Reports*, 1 (2012), 114–21.

19. Campagne DM, "The premenstrual syndrome revisited," *European Journal of Obstetrics & Gynecology and Reproductive Biology*, 130/1 (2007), 4–17.

6. How to be more active

1. Redman LM et al., "Metabolic and behavioral compensations in response to caloric restriction: implications for the maintenance of weight loss," *PLoS One* 4, e4377 (2009).

2. Garrow JS et al., "Meta-analysis: effect of exercise, with or without dieting, on the body composition of overweight subjects," *European Journal of Clinical Nutrition*, 49 (1995), 1–10.

3. Gill JM et al., "Exercise and postprandial lipid metabolism: an update on potential mechanisms and interactions with high-carbohydrate diets (review)," *The Journal of Nutritional Biochemistry*, 14/3 (2003), 122–32.

4. Byberg L et al., "Total mortality after changes in leisure time physical activity in 50 year old men: 35 year follow-up of population based cohort," *BMJ* 338 (2009), b688.

5. © Canadian Society for Exercise Physiology PAR-Q, www.csep.ca.

6. Wilmot EG et al., "Sedentary time in adults and the association with diabetes, cardiovascular disease and death: systematic review and meta-analysis," *Diabetologia* 55 (2012), 2895–2905.

7. Dunstan DW et al., "Breaking up prolonged sitting reduces postprandial glucose and insulin responses," *Diabetes Care*, 35/5 (2012), 976–83.

8. O'Donovan et al., "The ABC of Physical Activity for Health: a consensus statement from the British Association of Sport and Exercise Sciences," *Journal of Sports Sciences*, 28/6 (2010), 573–91.

9. King NA et al., "Individual variability following 12 weeks of supervised exercise: identification and characterization of compensation for exercise-induced weight loss," *International Journal of Obesity*, 32 (2008), 177–84.

10. Ainsworth BE et al., "2011 Compendium of Physical Activities: a second update of codes and MET values," *Medicine and Science in Sports and Exercise*, 43/8 (2011), 1575–81.

11. Ismail I et al., "A systematic review and meta-analysis of the effect of aerobic vs. resistance exercise training on visceral fat," *Obesity Reviews*, 13/1 (2012), 68–91.

12. Brinkworth GD et al., "Effects of a low carbohydrate weight loss diet on exercise capacity and tolerance in obese subjects," *Obesity* (Silver Spring), 17/10 (2009), 1916–23.

13. Farah NM et al., "Effects of exercise before or after meal ingestion on fat balance and postprandial metabolism in overweight men," *British Journal of Nutrition* (Oct. 26, 2012), 1–11.

7. How to stay slim

1. Sumithran P et al., "Long-term persistence of hormonal adaptations to weight loss," *The New England Journal of Medicine*, 365/17 (2011), 1597–1604.

2. Baldwin KM et al., "Effects of weight loss and leptin on skeletal muscle in human subjects," *The American Journal of Physiology—Regulatory, Integrative and Comparative Physiology*, 301/5 (2011), R1259–R1266.

3. Hall KD et al., "Quantification of the effect of energy imbalance on bodyweight," *The Lancet*, 378/9793 (2011), 826–37.

Appendixes

1. Gomez-Ambrosi J, Silva C, Catalan V et al., "Clinical usefulness of a new equation for estimating body fat," *Diabetes Care*, 35/2 (2012), 383–88.

2. Shea JL, King MT, Yi Y et al., "Body fat percentage is associated with cardiometabolic dysregulation in BMI-defined normal weight subjects," *Nutrition, Metabolism & Cardiovascular Diseases*, 229 (2012), 741–47.

3. Henry Basal CJK, "Metabolic rate studies in humans: measurement and development of new equations," *Public Health Nutrition*, 8/7a (2005), 1133–52.

4. Krieger JW et al., "Effects of variation in protein and carbohydrate intake on body mass and composition during energy restriction: a meta-regression," *The American Journal of Clinical Nutrition* 83/2 (2006), 260–74.

5. http://huhs.harvard.edu/assets/file/ourservices/service_nutrition_fiber.pdf.

6. *Plant Fiber in Foods*, 2nd ed., 1990. (HCF Nutrition Research Foundation Inc., PO Box 22124, Lexington, KY 40522).

acknowledgments

Many thanks to Anne Montague, Jo Godfrey Wood, and Mary Pegington for editing the manuscript; Kate Santon and Emily Jonzen for devising the recipes; Paula Stavrinos for her recipe ideas; and Kath Sellers for analyzing and collating the recipes for the book. Thanks also to Debbie McMullan and Rebecca Dodd-Chandler for their advice and expertise for the exercise chapter and to the illustrator, Stephen Dew.

This book has evolved from our research to date on intermittent diets for weight loss and reducing the risk of disease. We therefore thank our collaborators and colleagues who have made this work possible. First Mark Mattson from the National Institute on Aging, Baltimore, and Margot Cleary from the University of Minnesota for sharing the insights from their research, which inspired us to under-take our dietary studies. Second, the team of scientists and researchers who have helped us run these studies: Gareth Evans, Claire Wright, Ellen Mitchell, Helen Sumner, Rose-mary Greenhalgh, Jenny Affen, and Jayne Beesley at the Nightingale Centre and Genesis Breast Cancer Preven-tion. We are grateful to the rest of Mark Mattson's team, including Bronwen Martin and Roy Cutler, Jan Frystyk and Alan Flyvbjerg (Arhus University Hospital, Denmark), Roy Goodacre, Andrew Vaughan, Will Allwood, Robert Clarke, Kath Spence (all University of Manchester), Andy Sims (University of Edinburgh), and Wendy Russell (Rowett Institute), who have all helped to assess the impact of the diets on the body and disease risk. Thanks also to the following individuals for their invaluable advice: Susan Jebb (weight management), Julie Morris (statistics), and Louise Donnelly (health psychology and dieting behaviors).

Our greatest thanks are to Lester Barr, Pam Glass, and the Genesis Breast Cancer Prevention trustees, who have consistently supported our dietary research for the past 11 years. Also Nikki Hoffman, Michelle Cohen, the Genesis office team, and the Genesis volunteers who give up their time to help us in the office and run research clinics, particularly Jane Eaton, Susan Roe, Pauline Sadler, Philippa Quirk, Louise Blacklock, Alison Rees, and Angela Foster. Thanks also to Amy Tao and Matthew Collier, our Genesis graduate interns.

We thank the numerous dieters who have worked with us on the studies over the past 11 years, without whom none of the research would be possible, and staff within the Nightingale Centre and Genesis Breast Cancer Prevention who have been successfully dieting with our 2-Day Diet and inspired us to write this book.

Finally, Susanna Abbott and Catherine Knight at Ebury for their patience and hard work in making this book.

index

About the authors

Dr. Michelle Harvie and Professor Tony Howell work at the Genesis Breast Cancer Prevention Centre, part of the University Hospital of South Manchester NHS Foundation Trust. Genesis Breast Cancer Prevention is the only breast cancer charity in the UK entirely dedicated to prevention. Because weight is a significant factor in the risk of developing breast cancer, Dr. Harvie and Prof. Howell have spent years researching and developing the optimum diet to help people lose weight quickly and easily as well as keep off weight lost in the longer term. This incredibly effective diet is the result of their clinical research.

Dr. Michelle Harvie is an award-winning research dietitian. For the last 17 years she has specialized in optimum diet and exercise strategies for weight loss and preventing breast cancer and its recurrence. Her findings have been published in many major scientific journals. She was awarded the British Dietetic Association Rose Simmonds Award for best published dietetic research in 2005; Manchester City Council's 2007 International Women's Day Award for Women in Science; and the National Association for the Study of Obesity Best Practice Award for best published obesity research in 2010.

Professor Tony Howell is Professor of Medical Oncology at the University of Manchester. He has specialized in treating breast cancer for over 30 years and now focuses on pharmacological and lifestyle measures to prevent breast cancer. He is Research Director of Genesis Breast Cancer Prevention and has published over 600 scientific papers and book chapters, mainly concerning the biology of the breast and the treatment and prevention of breast cancer.

All author proceeds from the sale of this book will go to Genesis Breast Cancer Prevention (registered charity number 1109839), www.genesisuk.org.